YOUR AGELESS ATHLETE:

Training for Life

Charles Matthews

authorHOUSE®

AuthorHouse™
1663 Liberty Drive
Bloomington, IN 47403
www.authorhouse.com
Phone: 1 (800) 839-8640

Published by AuthorHouse 09/24/2016

ISBN: 978-1-5246-2396-8 (sc)
ISBN: 978-1-5246-2395-1 (e)

Print information available on the last page.

CONTENTS

INTRODUCTION

When I was a young child, I had asthma, which prevented me from doing anything athletic since even the smallest exertion caused me to wheeze and have shortness of breath. While I outgrew the asthma, I went through my teens, twenties, thirties, and half my forties without doing anything athletic to speak of. I had no athletic passions, nor any other real passions for that matter. In a word, I was miserable most of the time. Then I found my Ageless Athlete and everything changed. Beginning with small steps of athletic activity, my athletic passion grew, first for running and then for triathlons. This passion then carried over into other aspects of my life, and today I can happily say I have a passion for life.

Living as an Ageless Athlete is now part of my core being, and how that Ageless Athlete thinks and acts benefits all other aspects of my life. This book is about my journey from an unhappy, fat, out-of-shape, middle-aged man to the relatively fit and joyful athlete. You can discover your Ageless Athlete and your passion for life, as well, simply by following the steps I took.

This book is not about exercising, eating right, or giving up smoking, although these are all good things you may want to pursue as a result of reading this book. Certainly many competent and educated people have provided us with libraries of books on those subjects. This book, however, is about becoming an athlete at any age, but particularly if you're over 40, and reaping the broad-reaching, life-altering benefits of developing this deep-rooted part of ourselves. We are all athletes, and discovering this athleticism can change how we see ourselves, how we behave, and how we view life. Each of us can discover our athletic passion, whether it be competing in triathlons (like me), mountain climbing, hunting, kayaking, fishing, or even bowling, ping pong, or shooting pool. The task at hand is to find our Ageless Athlete, bring him or her into the sunlight, let him or her find an athletic passion, then train, and let him or her excel. As I hope to show you, the effects of understanding and developing your inner athlete can lead to a new and more positive attitude and view of yourself in practically all areas of your life.

I am over 60 years old as I write this book, which is based on my experiences and observations over approximately the past 20 years. It is aimed, therefore, at those in their middle years or older, who have been through the ropes of life for a while, have some rope burn, and may not show quite the same vigor as the younger generations. So I am not going to talk about the athletics of youth. Young athletes have their own place, but it is not in this book. I want to talk to and about middle-aged and older average people. Whether you were a competitive athlete in your younger years, or whether you were only a spectator, my journey will show you how to develop (or rekindle) your athleticism now. I want to help you find your Ageless Athlete. I want you to have a passion for life.

Did you know that, with just 12 weeks of standard strength training, we can stimulate and train "old" muscles to perform almost as well as they did when they were significantly younger? Exercise physiologists discovered and verified this fact by studying the muscles of sedentary people as old as 70. While the training process for a 70-year-old is certainly slower and less aggressive than it would be for a 30-year-old, people who couldn't get out of a chair without help are now able to climb stairs, carry packages, go for walks, and once again participate in life independently. They feel alert, vital and proud. Their newly cultivated "athleticism" has given them both a new physique and a new outlook on life. Newly born 70-year-old Ageless Athletes!

Did you know there is a Senior Olympics, too? The competitors are 50 and older, not so famous, not so fast and not so strong as those who compete in the Olympics we all know, but they are still athletes competing in a wide variety of individual and team events including badminton, basketball, bowling, golf, hockey, racquet ball, softball, cycling, track and field, swimming, running, volleyball, tennis, and even shuffleboard, horseshoes, and table tennis.

As I am sure you know, millions of baby boomers my age, as well as people who are both younger and older than I am, sit in front of televisions, computers, telephones, desks and windows every day, inactive, unmotivated, and, needless to say, often miserable in their daily lives. I know all about them. I used to be one of them. I, probably like many of you, never believed I could be anything else. I never knew I had any untapped athletic abilities or how powerful they could be. Lighting a cigarette or walking to the vending machine for a candy bar was as much athleticism as I exerted.

I'm living proof that becoming an athlete can happen at any age, and it can be fun, rewarding and life altering. I don't expect you to believe me at this point. I don't even expect you to want to do any kind of athletic training right now. But by the time you finish this little book, I not only hope to make you a believer, I also hope to make you a doer.

I want you to find your Ageless Athlete and discover the kind of athlete he or she wants to be. This means finding the athletic passion inside you. Then I want you to learn how to train your Ageless Athlete to achieve your passion and watch him or her excel far beyond any beliefs or expectations you may now have. Finally, I want you to see how your Ageless Athlete has become a part of you and *is* you in all areas of your life. In so doing, I promise you will find happiness, joy, and freedom in your daily living that you never experienced before.

But let's not get ahead of ourselves. You won't believe me anyway. You want proof? Well, read what happened to me.

PART A

MY JOURNEY

CHAPTER ONE — BUT I'M NOT EVEN ATHLETIC

Part 1: My Asthmatic Unhappy Childhood

At night, I cried to my mother that I could not breathe. I lied on my back, my side, my stomach, but I still gasped for air. I felt like I was going to die. I was frightened. My mother got out the air humidifier and rubbed Vicks on my chest to open the lung passages. Sometimes it helped. Sometimes it didn't. This routine didn't happen every night, but I never knew which nights it would happen. I was afraid to go to bed and I was always tired.

When I was a little older, the doctor prescribed a spray inhaler — a lifesaver — because it always opened my lungs when I wheezed. But the effect only lasted a short while and I couldn't take it too often. So sometimes I just tried to endure the wheezing. I took short breaths. I stayed perfectly still. I tried to remain calm. Needless to say, I couldn't do anything strenuous and certainly nothing particularly athletic. I loved to ride my bike between asthma attacks but sometimes an attack occurred while I was out riding and I was afraid to go any further than around the block for fear I wouldn't be able to get back. I saw other kids riding all over the neighborhood. I saw them playing ball, tag, or hide and seek. I wished I could play, too.

Later, when I was in high school, to be cool like the other kids I started smoking. Me, the asthmatic kid, inhaling cigarettes. By this time, my asthma attacks were rare, even though I still had my handy inhaler, and I still couldn't do anything too strenuous. I tried to play basketball and football with the neighborhood kids, but I couldn't run very far because I became winded and tired too quickly. So most of the time, I was just there watching, wanting to play, but unable. At school, I got this crazy idea to try out for (of all things) the track team. I did have these very muscular legs and was quite fast for 25 to 50 yards, so I thought perhaps I could be a sprinter or quarter miler. But with the shortness of breath I still experienced, I couldn't build up the stamina to do enough running in training to be fast enough to compete. So I switched to the shot put — a 5'6" kid weighing 140 pounds trying to throw a 12-pound shot put in competition with other kids one-and-a-half times bigger than I was. That didn't last long. So I stuck with academics and cigarettes and gave up sports. I wasn't happy but I was a really good student since I had all the time in the world to study and I didn't know how to do anything else. I excelled academically but still felt incomplete. This lifestyle carried right through my college and law school years.

As a lawyer, nothing changed. I worked hard, commuted to New York City from the suburban town where I grew up, got married, had two kids, and watched TV every night. I tried to work out at a gym occasionally, but since I had no passion or goals, I'd quit as soon as something interfered such as working late in the evening or sleeping late the next morning. I wasn't motivated to do anything except my dull routine, and I was only motivated to do that because I had to. That was my dreary life from my twenties to my early forties. I had no athletic activities and certainly no passion for anything going on in my life.

Part 2: My Ironman Triathlon

I was 54 years old. It was 8 p.m on a clear evening in July. I was in Germany and I had one mile to go in my Ironman triathlon. By this point in the race, my legs felt like they were running in mud. The mud turned to cement, and my legs to spaghetti. I started to imagine that someone slipped weights into my shoes when I wasn't looking. The swim, which started at 7 that morning, seemed like a century ago, but actually, it was more than a century. In bicycling parlance, a century is a 100-mile ride, and I had completed 112 after I finished the swim. But, oh that bike ride! A crowd of 1,000 enthusiastic spectators gathered at this hill in a small town in the middle of the German Black Forest countryside. They lined the sides of the road screaming encouraging exhortations of "whoosh, whoosh" in our ears as they parted to let our bikes through while we arduously climbed the hill. Other spectators called out our names as we passed, and saluted us with their steins of beer. I felt like a rider in the Tour de France!

But that was hours before the aching in the legs, the exhaustion, and the discouragement. I had already finished another quarter-century (25 miles) of the marathon run (with some walking along the way — I'm only human). The run course was actually marked in kilometers, 42 of them, and the distance between each seemed endless. What was I thinking when I thought I could do this? What was my wife thinking when she suggested we both do it as part of a European vacation? Some vacation — touring a canal from in the water, biking all over a hilly countryside, and then running along another part of that same canal just to be able to turn around at 13.1 miles and run back.

I was exhausted. I couldn't even feel my feet hitting the ground anymore. I wasn't even sure my legs would continue to move. Then I heard something along the sides of the road, first faintly, then gradually louder:

"You're almost there."
"You can do it."
"Don't give up."

It was the crowd cheering us on. Then it dawned on me: they believed in me. They wanted me to finish.

I was still on the course five hours after the overall race winner crossed the finish line. No matter. I wasn't there to win, but I had to find some way of ignoring the burning and numbness in my muscles. I had to keep going, so I thought of what I was accomplishing and the fact that I was nearing the end of this terrible labor of pain and, yes I'll say it, of love.

Only half a mile left. Thirteen hours and nine minutes down and about five minutes to go, but who's counting? I was going to finish this thing — running, not walking. Then I heard a low roar in the distance. It was the stadium crowd. I couldn't see the stadium at that point, but I knew I would get there, still standing.

The roar grew louder — like the deafening roar in a football stadium as the home team scored a touchdown. The big clock below the banner that sat over the finish line needlessly reminded me how long a day it had been. Most important, though, was the message the banner relayed: "Ironman Europe Finish." Was I dreaming or was I just delirious from dehydration and fatigue? No, I was about to go under it. Just a few more feet to go. The clock said 13:14:46, a time ever frozen in my mind, my time — the time of an Ironman Europe finisher!

I just had to figure out how to pose for the finish line picture. Hands clasped in prayerful thanks to God? Drop and kiss the ground? That was how I felt, but I thought it was probably too corny, and I probably wouldn't be able to get up again anyway. How about an arm pump and a Marv Albert "YES! YES!"

With 2.4 miles of swimming, 112 miles on my trusty bike, and 26.2 miles of running (and walking, but no crawling), I completed the Ironman Triathlon in Roth, Germany — my one and only Ironman! What a way to spend a summer vacation.

A thick red ribbon circled my sweaty neck and supported the Ironman finisher medal that rested in the middle of my chest. It was big and heavy and shaped like a number one, which meant we were all winners, and "Ironman Finisher" was inscribed on it in gold. To me, it felt like a Congressional Medal of Honor or, more appropriately, a Purple Heart. But it was now mine; I'd earned it, and I never wanted to take it off!

My wife, Patty, hugged me and said, "You're an Ironman!"

"Yes I am, and you are, too," I replied, as I felt the impression of her medal against my chest. She smiled. She finished about 20 minutes ahead of me. (Darn, I really wanted to beat her, but in a way I did. After all, I stayed out there longer than she did!)

I became an Ironman Finisher that day (I had to say it to myself a few times before it sank in). I received a finisher polo shirt, too — probably the hardest-earned piece of clothing I will ever have — and I joined an elite group of which only .00005% of the world's population were members. Pretty cool! Who would have thought I would ever be competing in an Ironman Triathlon, let alone at age 54?

Don't you remember? I was not athletic. I was the kid who, in the neighborhood baseball games, got sent out in right field where no one ever hit the ball (except that one time when a fly ball came toward me and I put my glove up to catch it — and it hit me in the head). I was the child with asthma who wheezed for dear breath from any physical exertion, and sometimes from none at all, the guy who the army wouldn't even take during the Vietnam War. I was the fellow who was 30 pounds overweight in law school and lived in the lunchroom between classes. How could I ever do anything athletic, let alone an Ironman? The answer: I became an Ageless Athlete!

Part 3: How I Discovered My Ageless Athlete

Let me take you back about 10 years earlier than my Ironman. One morning in May, I was having my morning cup of coffee with my first cigarette of the day. Even though I'd managed to lose 10 pounds since law school (thanks to stress), I was still a 44-year-old attorney, who was overweight by 20 pounds and smoking more than a pack of cigarettes a day. At the time, I'd been an attorney for almost 20 years, but I didn't enjoy the profession most of the time. I didn't know where my life was going or, for that matter, where it had gone. At that point, I had been in therapy for over nine years, but I was still depressed. If my life had continued that way, I would surely have been a candidate for death by alcohol, drugs or suicide, or, at the very least, I would have been sewing pretty moccasins or braiding lanyard key chains in a psycho ward. I felt like I was slipping away, sinking slowly into a bottomless pit, and didn't know how to make my life any better.

Suddenly the cigarette tasted bitter, so I put it out. Then, out of the drone of my depression, I heard a faint little voice in my head. Perhaps it had been there before and I just ignored it. It was barely more than a whisper but it grabbed my attention. I didn't know exactly why I was listening — maybe because I had reached the end of some invisible rope. The voice was not giving me any complex and overwhelming message about where my life was headed. It simply told me that, even if I were stuck in perpetual mediocrity, I could at least get a little bit healthier so my shirt buttons didn't pop at my waist and I stopped wheezing in my sleep. Even if I didn't feel in control of many things in my life, at least I could do something about my appearance and my health. After all, I stopped drinking nine months prior, so I felt I was at least beginning to improve my life.

The little voice dared to go on: Maybe I should work on a way to give up cigarettes. I had to admit it did seem somewhat inconsistent that I was trying to better myself mentally and emotionally, and yet I was still putting toxic smoke and chemicals into my lungs and body. Plus, even in high school when I started smoking, the cigarettes always had that bitter taste and burned my lungs. So, why not give quitting a try? Little did I know then that this urging inner voice was my Ageless Athlete, who was about to change my life dramatically.

My challenge was to give up smoking gradually (why be hasty after all?) while trying not to add to my already-expanded mid-body spare tire. I'd read the studies that showed my body was not absorbing 25 percent of my nutritional intake when I smoked. What a Catch-22! If I didn't give up smoking, my weight would remain the same but I would surely die of lung cancer or a stroke. But because I was giving up smoking, I'd gain weight since I'd be absorbing 25 percent more calories even if I didn't eat more and then I'd risk getting diabetes or dying from the effects of obesity. And of course those calories would join the settlement at my waist and I really couldn't afford more overcrowding there. A new fat wardrobe would have been quite expensive.

I was left with little choice. I had to figure out a way to occupy my non-smoking time with something that burned calories. I remembered the last time I gave up smoking, 17 years prior, but it only lasted until I got divorced seven years later and moved to the smoking capital of the East, New York City. During that smoke-free spell, I turned to running occasionally and it was actually fun at times. I recall running the two-mile loop from home to downtown and back a few days a week trying to get faster and faster and actually seeing improvement. I also dieted like crazy in a Quixotic quest to rid the world of my love handles. No ice cream except on weekends, healthy meats and vegetables for dinner during the week, and oh those lunchtime yogurts. Maybe I could do that again. It certainly made me feel better.

Recovery support groups have this idea of "one day at a time," which actually works pretty well. So I decided to give it a shot with smoking. I also learned as part of the recovery process that a person needed to change "people, places, and things" or run the risk of relapse. So I became a recovering smoker. Deep down, I came to believe that I was really a non-smoker who had been on the wrong path. I remembered how much I disliked the first morning cigarette but felt compelled to take it anyway. I remembered how I felt after being sick for a few days once and foregoing cigarettes until I was better. I felt good from that short smoking hiatus, but I didn't see enough compelling good coming from it to stay away. I was caught in a lifestyle where smoking seemed like one of my few pleasures, annoying as it was at times.

Over the first three weeks of my smoking recovery, I gradually cut down to five cigarettes a day. I gave up the cigarette with the first cup of coffee in the morning and started with the second cup. I cut out the cigarettes in the car. This actually improved my driving since I was no longer distracted trying to flick the ashes out the small crack in the car window or reaching under the steering wheel or on the seat between my legs for the dropped lit cigarette that was about to burn a hole in the floor mat, car seat or my pants. I also imposed a matches-out smoking curfew of 9 p.m., which gave me some great nights' sleep since I went to bed early because of the curfew.

While I cut back on the smokes, I added in physical activity. It started out as nervous pacing around my office with my hand anxiously going to my mouth so I could suck in and puff out air from my imaginary cigarette. Then, to avoid wearing out my shoe soles, I bought a pair of athletic running shoes (they used to be called sneakers before their price skyrocketed) and commenced fast walking outside with intermittent spurts of slow running. Gradually, the running spurts got longer and I was up to a half mile without stopping. I won't say it was an easy transition. It took many battles in my head to motivate my legs. I had to constantly fight against the inner exhortations to go watch TV instead of going out the door. But with each walk and run, the endorphins released from my brain gave me deep feelings of calmness and well being — and even fleeting feelings of happiness and a sense of accomplishment. I always felt better after exercising than I did before.

Then that little voice inside gave me another nudge: "When you stop smoking completely, why don't you train for a short local race?"

This time I answered back: "What, are you crazy? Me, a runner — in a race? You've got to be kidding! I'd never make it and I hate the idea of being last and all alone." In my mind, I was still the asthmatic, uncoordinated, sedentary child who'd smoked since high school.

But the voice kept repeating the question and, with much fear and trepidation, I signed up for a 5K (3.1 mile) running race taking place later in the summer in a local town park where at least a thousand other people would be running. I figured that was my best chance to get lost in the crowd and hopefully (and most importantly) not come in alone and last. I did not want to feel that humiliation and I hadn't yet learned that someone is always last and the real loser is the person who does not finish at all. Years later I actually came in last in a swimming race and, while I wasn't thrilled about it, I wasn't devastated either and now I can even laugh about it. A month before the race, I was running about a mile non-stop and still smoking a few cigarettes each day, more out of fear of ending the habit than out of pleasure — like wanting to hold onto a friend who was about to move away. I set May 14, two weeks before the race, as my last smoking day, and I held to it. Today, all these years later, I still have my last empty cigarette pack from that day as a reminder and memento of my accomplishment. I even consider it a trophy.

I gradually increased my running, not just to prepare for the race, but also because I was a bundle of nerves and didn't know what to do with myself. But it worked! Race day came and there at the start was the famous Bill Rodgers, multiple New York City and Boston Marathon winner. He was a race icon and celebrity runner who led the pack (race officials told me he actually won, but I sure wasn't at the finish in time to see it). I was quite impressed just to be in the same park, let alone in the same race, with such an athlete.

One thousand of us, all shapes and sizes, gathered at the start in the parking lot of this beautiful park on Long Island Sound, crowding next to each other rows deep. Then bang! The gun went off and so did the runners. There were spectators lined all along the course cheering us on. I was so proud to be one of those they were cheering. I remember feeling strong and powerful as I took off, but I hadn't learned to pace myself. So, after the first half mile, my legs and lungs tired and running became increasingly difficult. And darned if they didn't put a couple of hills in the course just to annoy me. The first finishers crossed the finish line about 15 minutes after the start and the stream of human bodies continued for the next half hour. Then the crowds dispersed and darkness came in...and so did I. No, it wasn't that bad. I wasn't last or alone. I was somewhere in the second half of the finishers — safe, comfortable, and anonymous. I was more than 10 minutes slower than the first finishers but I felt a tremendous sense of pride and accomplishment. I ran hard, persevered, and crossed the finish line, and that made me a winner. For the first time in my life, I felt like an athlete. I cannot describe that feeling other than both cosmic and orgasmic at the same time. I was at one with my body and the world and it felt like I'd found a key part of my identity after a long, lonely search in a strange and hostile land. I felt exhilarated, safe, comfortable, and proud. I discovered my Ageless Athlete!

Part 4: My Ageless Athlete Grows

The series of events that followed in my life was nothing short of amazing. Within a year and a half after that first race, I completed the New York City Marathon, running side by side with my closest friend — a friendship that developed through our common interest in running and our shared belief that the physical, mental, and emotional states are closely intertwined. This is extraordinary for several reasons:

First, as I said, I had never been "athletic." For me as a kid, playing neighborhood baseball (what little I could do between asthma attacks) was the frightful and humiliating experience of striking out constantly while trying to get a walk (I knew I'd never be able to hit that little ball) and praying no one hit the ball to me in right field. Playing neighborhood football was something I ardently avoided like the plague. In those instances where peer pressure made playing unavoidable, it meant running for dear life if I got the football so I wouldn't be tackled by the bigger guys and, on defense, trying not to be near the guy with the football so I wouldn't get hurt trying to tackle him. I did like to ride my bike, but because of my unpredictable asthma attacks, I was afraid to ride very long or far from home. On some days, the end of the driveway seemed like all I could handle. As I got older, the asthma subsided, but by then I was driving a car (and my bike had been stolen anyway). So, to train for and run 26.2 miles through the streets of New York City, with millions of live and television spectators, was never even in the remotest of my dreams or lifetime possibilities.

Second, I was always quiet, shy and reclusive and had never been good at developing friendships, particularly male friendships, so a "jock" friend and training buddy was absolutely unheard of. Then to actually run the full marathon with this guy by my side for mutual support and camaraderie was unthinkable.

Third, I didn't particularly believe in God, order in the universe, or anything positive in the world. So, to develop a sense of cosmic and personal integration, self-esteem, fitting in as part of a larger picture, and just feeling happy and connected were not only new, but shocking, experiences for me. I actually stopped feeling depressed.

Then, my new-found Ageless Athlete suggested I could have an additional career mission beyond being a lawyer. So I entered a Master's program in Exercise Physiology at a local university so I could learn how the body functions and how physical training is accomplished. I learned about how so much of the aging process can be slowed down and many of its effects even reversed through simple athletic activities like walking, swimming, cycling and a little weight training. I became acquainted with the mind-body connection and the importance of physical activity in alleviating depression. I already knew firsthand how feeling and looking better physically improved my sense of self-esteem and self-worth, but I came to understand better the myriad of ways our Ageless Athletes can make that happen.

With this new-found knowledge, I became a certified personal trainer and started doing hands-on training for others like me. I saw my trainees get healthier physically, mentally, and emotionally. I saw the awakening of their Ageless Athletes and the positive personalities and lifestyle changes that followed. They were happier and thanked me for it, but I was just a messenger for their Ageless Athletes.

I even remarried — to Patty — a woman who shares my love of and belief in the importance of athletic training as a part of life at any age. She, too, gave up smoking (after being relegated to the garage and winter cold for her cigarettes since I had become the epitome of the intolerant reformed smoker). Then she picked up running, and several years later, we had the once-in-a-lifetime thrill of running the 100th Boston Marathon, crossing the finish line hand in hand (with a picture to prove it). Patty also became a personal trainer. We were married one sunny August afternoon on the beach in Florida — she in her beautiful white dress with white pumps, and I in my tuxedo with white and gold running shoes I purchased especially for the occasion. I was so nervous the day of the wedding that I ran 10 miles up and down the beach to try and calm down. It almost worked (and I didn't smoke).

Today, I am still a lawyer, but not at the same workaholic levels (I do enough to cover the bills, savings, vacations, training equipment, and race-entry fees) and I enjoy it much more than I used to. I also derive a tremendous sense of satisfaction from helping other men and women discover their Ageless Athletes, feel better, and improve the quality of their lives. They all appreciate it, which is a reward in itself. While I generally don't compete in marathons anymore, I now compete in triathlons (swim, bike, run) and love calling myself a triathlete. The Ironman was the thrill of a lifetime, although, since having an arthritic hip replaced, I prefer the shorter so-called sprint-distance triathlons (less wear and tear on the body and more time for other life interests) and I have even won some medals and prizes in my age group (when not too many others show up). I, the former klutz, can now do three athletic activities, and the training is never boring. Although I am by no means elite or more than moderately competitive in my age group, I'm still an athlete who has grown into a man who cares about himself and others and has a place and purpose in this world.

To sum up, I'm not a jogger and I don't exercise. *I'm an Ageless Athlete and I train!*

CHAPTER TWO — BUT I'M NOT COMPETITIVE

When I was a young boy and teenager, I often played ping pong with my friends, using our family ping pong table in the basement. In fact, I got to be pretty good at spins, hooks, and slams, and defensively very little got by me. In practice, I could hit everything and rarely missed. In a competitive game, however, I made silly mistakes and gave away points — especially late in the game. I probably lost more games than I won yet I was a more skilled player than most of my opponents. After a while, I gave up competing in ping pong and eventually gave up the sport entirely.

High school wasn't much different. In my freshman year, I ran track and was actually fairly fast for a short distance. But because of my lack of stamina, rather than continue to work at it, I switched to shot put. As I previously said, me, at 140 pounds and 5'6", trying to throw a 12-pound steel ball in competition with guys almost twice my size. I soon gave that up and dedicated myself to smoking on the bus after school.

I forgave myself for my non-athleticism by saying that sports weren't that important and I wasn't the competitive type anyway. So I tried to get all A's in academics and not let anyone score higher than I did. So much for thinking I wasn't competitive. But of course I didn't see it at the time.

This "non-competitive" attitude carried right into my career where I clandestinely compared myself, my situations, and my accomplishments to those around me. While I didn't want anyone to think I was measuring them or competing with them, I was always focused on the hierarchical pecking order and the rewards each level offered. My self-worth was directly tied to my sense of position among others. Of course, this attempt to fill the inside with the outside was a doomed endeavor since, put simply, I was like a sieve and never satisfied. I always needed more and never felt like I was part of a team, let alone a co-member of the human race.

I can vividly remember working toward becoming a partner in the law firm where I was employed in New York. It took about seven years to be considered for partnership and I was in my seventh year. So was another attorney with whom I had gone to law school and developed a close friendship over the years. During that seventh year, I became distant from him, watching everything he did, making sure he was not trying to sabotage my partnership chances, wanting to show him up wherever I could, or at least not look less competent than he did. I made partnership my life's goal to the exclusion of all others, as if my entire self worth depended on winning this "award" of status. And, perhaps not so strangely since we came from similar backgrounds, he was doing the same with me. Two supposed friends, each battling with all our might to beat the other, lest our most important career goal be compromised. Our friendship fell by the wayside, and although we both made partner that year, we were never close again. Ironically, by six years later, we both had left the law firm for other legal employments. At the time, I didn't realize what a heavy price I paid for my overly competitive drive to achieve partnership status.

Although I functioned as if I "had it all together," I always thought of myself as different from others. I trusted nobody, made few friendships, and operated pretty much in my own world that seemed to have no purpose or happiness, notwithstanding the achievements and material possessions I obtained. While I appeared well off by most external measuring sticks, the very core of my personality was flawed and the result was an attitude of negativism that permeated my entire worldview. I now know that, as overly simplistic as it may sound, the lack of athletic activity in my life was a major contributor to my morose, my distrustful attitude, and my isolated existence. My clandestine and misplaced competitiveness was a symptom of a cancer that was destroying my spirit.

Aside from the physical health and well being that my Ageless Athlete has brought me, he has also given me a new outlook on life, a kind of meta-physical CPR — a cardio-pulmonary resuscitation where, through my athletic activities, the stimulation of my heart muscle (cardio) lets me see more goodness in the world (and even in other human beings). In addition, the expanded ability of my lungs (pulmonary) allows me to breathe in the nurturing fresh air of the natural harmony, balance, and order that exists in me and the world. Pretty lofty stuff. You don't have to buy it, but when I'm training, that's how I feel, and I feel good feeling that way. Maybe it's the endorphins released from the training that provide lasting calmness and satisfaction. Daily endorphin release is certainly better than daily cigarette smoking. Perhaps it's the mind-body connection that has led me to put aside my competitiveness and need to be better than others in my daily world. I now compete in an athletic field where I feel much more appropriate and fulfilled.

While I really don't know where this new me comes from, I do know it is a direct result of finding and training my Ageless Athlete. These days, even channeling my competitiveness to my athletic events is not so much a competition against others (although I do like the medals) as it is an internal competition to improve and progress. And I never lose because my Ageless Athlete has taught me not to quit and that crossing the finish line is always a winning proposition.

Most important, though, I learned a deeper message about handling life. My competitiveness had been misdirected, or maybe more accurately, it was scattered and improperly focused. Competitiveness was actually the way I expressed my aggressiveness and my desire for power, control, and recognition. The problem was I was using it in the wrong places and for the wrong purposes. Aggressiveness, power, control, and recognition are all athletic characteristics and motivators. Channeled properly in that direction, they can lead to immensely fulfilling and rewarding achievements. Channeled improperly, they can lead to anger, resentment, jealousy, and never being satisfied or having enough. After all, is the proverbial 15 minutes of fame really enough? Do we ever have enough toys? Isn't the grass always greener next door?

Don't get me wrong. We can all strive for material success, and it does provide a level of happiness and, perhaps equally important, a feeling of security. It isn't as secure as it seems, though, and happiness passes into boredom as well as a desire for the rush of more "happiness." A new balance in living will arise if we take a portion of the energy we put into material striving and give it to our Ageless Athletes. Every day I can put this energy into a specific training regimen where I can see a visible improvement in how I look, feel, and perform. Then I can feel the sense of pride and accomplishment that racing and finishing bring. And my fatigue comes not from the mental and emotional stress that used to plague me, but from using my muscles in a healthy way. Sure, my Ageless Athlete is competitive, but that's what athletes are and that's what they are supposed to be. I don't have to hide it anymore or try to limit it. My Ageless Athlete has given it an outlet that makes sense. I still want to compete at times when someone passes me on the interstate, but the feeling is short-lived because I don't want to injure my Ageless Athlete. I don't want to kill myself anymore. My life is just too much fun to give it up that way. Yours can be, too! Read on.

PART B

YOUR JOURNEY

CHAPTER THREE — NO EXCUSES

Before we delve into how you find, train and enjoy your Ageless Athlete, I would like to share a few more stories to put to rest some common excuses I often hear people give to avoid engaging in an athletic activity. Even if these are not your excuses, I think you will still find the stories interesting, educational, and even inspiring. Then we can get down to the business of how you create your own inspiring story.

Excuse 1: I'm Too Busy To Train (Orly's Story)

Orly is a friend of Patty's. She is a woman in her 40s, owns her own landscaping business, and has a husband and two young children. About four years ago, she decided she needed to lose some excess weight. Orly is 5'9" and played some athletics in her high school and college days, but running her business and attending to her family took its toll on her, both physically and emotionally. She was stressed, tired, and while she exercised at the health club a few times a week on a Nordic trainer, she had no other athletic interests or motivations and felt the little she was doing was not much benefit.

Orly knew my wife was a personal trainer and asked her for help. She started out with a little nutritional education, some additional aerobic exercises, and a couple of sessions per week of weight training. Then Orly's Ageless Athlete got involved. During the personal training sessions, Patty told

Orly about triathlons, and with a little prompting, Orly made a commitment to compete in a short one later that year. Patty worked up a triathlon training plan for Orly, and that year, Orly completed her first triathlon in Florida. A year later she finished a half-ironman distance triathlon and her smile across the finish line went from pole to pole. She also qualified to go to the world triathlon championships in her weight division. As I mentioned, Orly is a big woman and, as such, she qualified for the Athena athlete division, which is for those above certain weight levels, not necessarily because they're fat, but because they're bigger than average size. For men, this is called the Clydesdale athlete division. That's one of the beauties of triathlons (and certain other athletics) — they recognize both age group and size classifications.

Orly will probably never be as thin as a marathon runner because that's just not her body shape. But she could still run a marathon if she trained for it. Being an athlete is not limited to any particular size or shape. At my Ironman in Germany, for example, one of the finishers was a 35-year-old ex-football player weighing in excess of 300 pounds. When I saw him at the start, I couldn't believe anyone that big could even find a bike strong enough to hold him. I certainly didn't believe he would cycle 112 miles on it after a 2.4-mile swim and then run 26.2 miles, but he did it, and you would be amazed at the number of other triathlete men and women in the high weight divisions. But I digress.

Make no mistake, Orly put in numerous hours of training time to get to the levels she has achieved. My wife and I would go on many a bike ride with her only to hear a faint ringing sound and we would turn to see Orly clutching her cell phone to her ear on the side of the road because she needed to address a pressing business or family matter. But after the call, she was back in the saddle continuing her training ride, and when the ride was over and she went back to work, she was more relaxed and less stressed.

Orly has been able to develop a lifestyle where, during triathlon season (mostly summer), she can spend about eight to 10 hours a week swimming, biking, running, and weight training, in addition to working full time plus overtime running her business with her husband. Yet she also finds time to help their children with their homework, attend school functions, and be on the sidelines for soccer, baseball, football, and other extra-curricular activities. Orly is calmer, more organized, and much happier than she was before she found her Ageless Athlete, although she is obviously a busy lady. She says she now enjoys life to its fullest and marvels at how far her Ageless Athlete has taken her.

How did she do it, you ask? Well, Orly made a schedule. She started with the number of hours in a day (24) and then deducted the sleep she needed (in her case, seven hours). With the 17 remaining hours, she deducted her work hours (8 a.m. to 5 p.m. = 9 hours including lunch break). Then she deducted her dinner and evening time with her husband and children (6 p.m. to 10 p.m. = 4 hours). That left her four hours each day during the workweek to schedule her training, although she also had to make room for cheering her boys on in their athletics activities, church, PTA, and occasional unforeseen events requiring her attention.

So, with all her commitments, how was Orly able to fit in the right amount of training and not feel totally stressed out about it? By making her training a priority. Priority doesn't mean she ignored the rest of her required daily activities. It means she scheduled her training time so it fit into her daily activities and stuck to the schedule, which will sometimes mean re-arranging other activities. I'm sure this sounds like blasphemy to many of you, but you would be surprised how easy it is to keep to your training schedule and move something else around if training is your priority.

My training, much of which I do in the morning, has allowed me to function better in my other activities. Many a time, after a work-related, stress-induced, bad night's sleep, I've thought, *Gee, I'll have to skip training this morning to get to work early because I have so many things to do today,* but luckily, I end up feeling guilty and worrying that if I give in to it, I'll run the risk of skipping it repeatedly. This is how the mind works sometimes. So, after I've overcome that temptation, my next thought is, *Gee, getting my training in before work will allow me to be more productive and, if I have to work late, I can do that.* I have found the fear I have in the morning of not completing my work requirements for that day is the result of my mind feeling stress, and that fear is not necessarily real. I often project that something is going to take longer to complete than it actually does. I also need to measure how important getting to work early really is. Is it more important than my health and being true to my inner athletic self? Of course, during the times when work or some other activity must take precedence, I look to see if the training can fit in at another point during the day. If not, I let it go for that day and see if I can increase my physical activity during the other training sessions that week to account for the missed day.

For Orly to make her training a priority, she determined her Ageless Athlete was an early riser and therefore generally awoke at 5:30 a.m. to use the early hours as training time, before the daily chaos commenced. She was at the local pool by 6 a.m. for a swim three times during the week and did strength training the other two weekday mornings. Many a dark winter's morning would find her, barely awake with her cup of tea in hand, driving to the pool at her local Y, wearing a heavy coat over her bathing suit and carrying work clothes in her gym bag. And since misery loves company, she would cajole my wife into meeting her there for a workout.

Actually, that brings up a key training tip: Find a training partner with similar athletic interests. You may not need a partner at every session, but certain workouts every week could be a team effort. Plus, the support and camaraderie add a key element to your motivation, not to mention a bit of friendly competition as your partner encourages you to push harder. Also, when one of you wants to bag a workout, the other is there to keep it from happening. Guilt can be a great motivator.

Back to Orly. After the swim and a quick breakfast (very important), by 8 a.m. she was ready to start her work day. Since triathlon training involves three athletics, on most days Orly had two workouts of either biking or running three to four days each work week. Depending on the weather and her schedule, she added a bike ride or a run either during lunch, the hour before dinner after work, or in the evening on her indoor trainer in the basement while she was watching television after the children were asleep and while her husband was doing something else. She needed to be careful with these late evening bike rides, however, since her body was always so energized after a workout that she might find sleeping difficult if she didn't wait long enough for fatigue to set in before bedtime. So any late evening sessions were less intense than her other rides and were more like maintenance and recovery training. We will discuss these types of training in the chapter about how to train.

Although Orly's business and family activities were high priorities on the weekends, she tried to keep the hours between 6 a.m. and 10 a.m. available for the longer bike rides and runs. In the summer, going to the beach with her family also gave her an opportunity to squeeze in some outdoor swimming.

As you can see, Orly led a busy life before she started training for triathlons. But with the discipline and motivation her Ageless Athlete provided, she had plenty of time to train without feeling stressed. In fact the early morning training gave her a much calmer attitude, more energy for her other daily activities, increased ability to cope with all the stresses that arose during the day, and a sounder, more restful sleep in the evenings.

Most triathlons start between 6 and 7 a.m. on a Saturday or Sunday. For most triathletes, a full season of racing is relatively short and involves competing only once, sometimes twice, a month during the summer. Since Orly's races were generally local, she didn't have to travel far and could be back home by noon. If the race was near a beach or an amusement park, Orly would take her family, and they'd cheered her on at a race or two. For her Florida races (she competes in one triathlon each year in St. Petersburg), she'd add a couple of extra days so that she and her husband could enjoy a long weekend away together.

The point is, with a little prioritizing and creative thinking, Orly was able to add a sport that required a significant amount of training, without losing the levels of involvement and dedication she put into her business and family — all without an increase in stress level or fatigue. To this day, she gets plenty of sleep; eats balanced meals; is a resourceful boss, loving wife, and dedicated mother; and has an Ageless Athlete who brings her a deep, personal physical and mental satisfaction and a healthy lifestyle. As a result, she stands a better chance of continuing to be effective in all her roles for a very long time than she did before she started training. Plus she is setting a good example for her children of how becoming athletes can lead to happy, balanced, and productive lives. And all of this started because Orly wanted to lose weight and get in better shape. It's truly wondrous how our Ageless Athletes can get our attention and change our lives.

Excuse 2: I'm Not Healthy Enough To Train (John's Story)

John was diagnosed with AIDS. That's what the doctors told him. Today they're not sure anymore, though, because his blood count has been normal for more than a year. Just two-and-a-half years ago, John didn't expect to live long and wanted to do something unusual and fulfilling before he died — something his family and friends would remember and appreciate. Seemingly out of nowhere, his Ageless Athlete suggested an absolutely preposterous idea: *why not do an Ironman Triathlon?* John was taken aback but intrigued by the thought. For whatever reason (and I would say it was the inner voice of his Ageless Athlete), John decided to do it.

Not quite understanding why he was doing it, whether he could finish it, or even whether he could handle the rigorous training process, he began to train. While John was somewhat athletic in his younger years (some team athletics in high school, a little golf and tennis, and an occasional bike ride or trail run), he had not engaged in much physical activity since his diagnosis. About nine months before the Ironman race, the doctors told him they weren't sure if he had enough time left, let alone enough stamina to go through with it. But John was convinced that this was the feat he wanted to be remembered for, and that he could pass on a message to others with AIDS that they should strive to live their lives to the fullest regardless of how long they had left and regardless of their physical condition. It took John weeks to build up the stamina just to do two short training sessions of the different disciplines in one day. But with every week that went by, John grew stronger physically and in his belief that his goal seemed more and more attainable. Gradually, he continued his training process, adding more double sport training days, then increasingly longer workouts, and even some speed work at the track. In spite of his disease, John was becoming an athlete and he loved the feeling. His doctor was skeptical about the effects the triathlon would have on John's body, but John told him he felt more alive, had a purpose, enjoyed what his body was doing, and could do so much to improve his fitness.

By the third month of training, the doctor couldn't deny that John was showing prodigious results. John applied for the Ironman Hawaii triathlon, which is the world championship triathlon event, only open to a select number of triathletes who have qualified through top finishes in specific qualifying races, with a limited number of lottery slots offered as well. John was nowhere near being sufficiently trained or physically gifted to qualify, but he could certainly enter the lottery. And since lottery entrants could include a short description of why they should be chosen for an entry slot, John explained his situation on his entry form, including what he had accomplished in his training as well as the message he wanted to convey to others with his condition. The Ironman Hawaii triathlon is nationally televised, and the race organizers decided John should be given the chance to compete. So they alerted the television media about him. If John was able to complete his training and start the race, regardless of whether he could finish, he would have the opportunity to show the world that being diagnosed with AIDS is not an immediate death sentence.

John was psyched. But then, about two months before his race, his father became very ill. John had not been close to his father for many years. Now, with this new development, and his own unknown future, he wanted to make amends for all the lost time. Even with John's increasingly longer Ironman training requirements, he started spending more time with his father. He wanted to give him the gift of being in Hawaii for the race and seeing him finish, although he feared his father might not make it. With this new impetus, John became even more dedicated that ever to his goal.

Well, John and his father both made it to Hawaii. It was somewhat ironic that John's father, who had been so physically strong all his life, was now frail and John, with his incurable and debilitating disease, was the strongest he had ever been. His father couldn't have been more proud of his son.

Race day started at 4 a.m. John got dressed, had an easily digestible nutritious breakfast, and went to the race site to make sure his bike was ready and his other transition items were properly in place. The race started at 6 a.m. when all 1,500 participants started to swim en masse. The winner finished in less than 9 hours. For John, the race was much longer — more than 16 hours — but he had enough energy left to hug his father at the finish line. John had completed his first Ironman Triathlon. I say first because he completed another one seven months later and was back at the Hawaii race a year later to complete his third.

But John's first Ironman is the one he cherishes most. He was not especially fast, but that didn't matter. He finished. His father, after a successful operation, was there for the other races as well and their relationship has become very close — all because of John's Ageless Athlete. John doesn't think so much about dying anymore, although he has long outlived some of his closest friends who also had AIDS. He now fits in well with his many new friends who are also triathletes and shares their vitality and enthusiasm for life. As he says, through his Ageless Athlete, he found his own empowerment, while his doctors are still scratching their heads about John's miraculous recovery.

Excuse 3: Is It Really Worth It?
(The Story of Team Hoyt)

I was participating in a triathlon a few years ago in a little out-of-the-way beach town called Barrington, Rhode Island. It was race morning and, as usual, everyone was nervously tinkering with their bikes, adjusting their wetsuits, or merely pacing around in anxious anticipation of the start.

As the race was about to get underway, the starter announced that, before the age group waves began, race officials would give a head start to a special couple from Massachusetts who came to compete. Their last name is Hoyt, and they are endearingly called "Team Hoyt." Ricky Hoyt was almost 40 years old at the time and is a paraplegic who cannot walk, move his hands, or talk. He communicates through slight head movements picked up by a keyboard on a computer attached to his wheelchair that allows him to "speak." Ricky loves competing in triathlons with his father, Dick.

At the time of the Barrington race, Dick Hoyt was in his 60s, slightly overweight, and not someone you would think of as a runner, let alone a swimmer and a cyclist. I certainly did not know at the time that Team Hoyt began in 1997, competing in a five-mile run. Actually, it was Ricky's idea to do that five-mile run because it was a benefit run for a local lacrosse player who became paralyzed in an accident. Dick pushed Ricky across the finish line in a wheelchair. They were next to last but the feeling of triumph overwhelmed any latent negative thoughts about where they finished. This magical moment woke up both their Ageless Athletes. As Ricky puts it, he just doesn't feel handicapped when he and his dad are competing. They went on to compete in more races over the next eight years and actually finished in the top quarter of the Boston Marathon. Then, in 1985, as a Father's Day present to his dad's Ageless Athlete, Team

Hoyt participated in its first triathlon, and the two of them have been triathletes ever since. They even completed the Ironman Triathlon in Hawaii.

So, on this day in Barrington, as the rest of us waited for our wave, Dick and Ricky prepared to start. Dick was standing hip deep in the water in his wetsuit, and wrapped around his waist were straps that attached to a small boat (yes, I said boat) in which Ricky sat. The gun went off and Dick started his half-mile swim, towing Ricky behind him. I watched in amazement only to learn later that, like me, Dick didn't know how to swim when Ricky decided they should try triathlons. And he hadn't biked since he was a kid.

With Team Hoyt well into their swim, the rest of the waves started and even I, a slow swimmer in a late wave, caught and passed Ricky and Dick. But that didn't matter to them. They just kept going.

Since the 13-mile bike course was an "out and back" course, meaning it was the same course going out and coming back, the bikers got to see one another on the return trip. As I was coming back, I caught a glimpse of Dick and Ricky. Dick was pedaling a specially made bike, with Ricky sitting in a basket-like contraption over the front wheel and attached to the handle bars. It is difficult enough for me to push my own, plus my bike's, weight up hills and against the wind. The aerobars attached to my handlebars allow me to be more aerodynamic and reduce the wind resistance and, my titanium bike weights less than 17 pounds. But I can't imagine how hard it must have been for Dick to balance the weight of a full-grown man on the front of his bike, let alone carry him through the course. But there they were, pedaling along at a competitive pace, with Dick nodding his head in appreciation to the cheering on-lookers and co-competitors.

I didn't see Dick and Ricky again until the end of the race when Dick, pushing Ricky in front of him in a specially made stroller, crossed the finish line after his 5K run. Their finishing time? Who knows and who cares. Certainly not Team Hoyt. They were all smiles and full of joy. After all, the run must have seemed like a breeze to Dick after many years of pushing Ricky in his heavy wheelchair through several marathons.

I later found out that Team Hoyt is famous in the triathlon world, not because of their blazing speed or endurance, but because of the love they share — the love of a father and son and the love of being athletes together. Whenever I start to think that maybe I should quit a race or, on a really bad day, the whole sport of triathlon, I think of Team Hoyt, my wife, and our triathlete friends. Like Ricky and Dick, my wife and I have a shared love for triathlons, and our triathlon friends give us a sense of belonging, as I am sure is the case for the Hoyts. That's one of the great rewards of participating in a sporting activity.

It wasn't always that way for the Hoyts, though. Before they started on their great adventure, Dick was a couch potato. On that notable day in 1997 when Ricky asked his father if they could do that five-mile benefit run together, Dick (with a significant amount of fear and second thoughts) said he would do it for Ricky. Ageless Athletes sometimes emerge from the most unexpected places. With every race they finished, Ricky's smile and happiness grew larger and Dick grew closer to his son. They trained together all the time. For the longer triathlons, Dick often trained up to five hours a day, five times a week, while still working his regular job. They traveled to races all around the country and abroad and saw places they never would have seen otherwise. They became inspirations to thousands of other budding athletes as well as some in their waning years. Some people approached them and said, "We just want to thank you; we're here because of you," While others thought, *Hey, look at those two! How can I complain about how tough it is on me?*

So, is it really worth it? You bet it is.

CHAPTER FOUR — WHO IS YOUR AGELESS ATHLETE? WHAT IS YOUR PASSION?

Athleticism is a fundamental characteristic of every living creature. A fish that swims through the water, then dives to eat algae off a rock, is engaging in athletic activity. A worm that inches its way over grass, then burrows into a dirt hole, is being athletic. A dog that chases a thrown Frisbee, then catches it in mid-air, is athletic. A horse that races through a field, then jumps over a stone wall or a brook, is exhibiting athletic abilities. A young child who runs after a soaring badminton birdie, then hits it with a racket (no matter where the birdie goes), is certainly behaving athletically. Even an old man casting his fishing line to just the right spot in the river, then getting a bite, and reeling in his catch is athletic. What then is athleticism? Put simply, it is the mind-body connection of using muscles in a purposeful way toward a decided goal. Whether the particular goal is achieved only defines how well a person has learned the athletic activity, not whether a person is athletic. Any athlete knows the benefits of being athletic — the feelings of well-being, contentment, and accomplishment. I know a prominent psychiatrist who puts it this way: athleticism is the poor man's Prozac.

So the first lesson to learn from all I have said up to now is this: if you have a mind and a body and can exert some purposeful use of both together, *you are an athlete*, no matter what your age. Verbalizing this simple, yet powerful, truth helped me become an Ageless Athlete. At first, all I could do was express this concept in the third person, like I was talking to myself from the outside. I would say:

"YOU ARE AN ATHLETE, AN AGELESS ATHLETE!"

Then I internalized it by taking a deep breath, and saying out loud:

"I AM AN ATHLETE, AN AGELESS ATHLETE."

As I said it, I actually started feeling stronger and more self-assured. I raised my chin, put my shoulders back, and said it again. Repeating it louder and stronger became one of my first training exercises:

"I AM AN ATHLETE, AN AGELESS ATHLETE."

Finally, I began to believe it and my mantra became:

"I AM AN AGELESS ATHLETE."

Amazingly, from this simple repetition, I started to feel in my heart and gut that I AM an Ageless Athlete, not because of my current physical condition, but because of the drive inside me to train my body to match what my mind was thinking. Being an Ageless Athlete is an element of who I am — of who we all are. By realizing this truth in your mind first and then training your body to match your thoughts, a sense of power will come over you as it did for me, and your Ageless Athlete will emerge. Try it. Stop reading, put this book down, stand up, and say out loud a few times:

"I AM AN ATHLETE, AN AGELESS ATHLETE."

Enjoy the tingling this sense of power creates in you. Strut around if the urge strikes you. Walk like an athlete with your head up, shoulders back, chest out, and stomach in (even if it doesn't look like it's in). Notice the muscles in the back of your neck that let you lift your chin, the back muscles that contract when you put your shoulders back and your chest out, and the abdominal muscles working as you suck in your stomach. You can control and direct your muscles using thought commands. What marvelous creatures we are that we can do these things!

The next step for me was to think bigger. I needed an athletic passion that would allow me to work all of my major muscle groups. That led me to think about competing in a triathlon. A friend of mine at work mentioned he competes in a short triathlon once a year, so I thought to myself, *Hey, if he can do it, why can't I?* So I dusted off my old bicycle I bought 15 years earlier to take my son for rides on Sundays. Next I joined the local Y to learn how to swim, and finally I started training. I had no idea whether I could do a triathlon, but I liked the idea of learning how to swim and getting back on a bike, though I won't go into the details of those early training months (yes, *months*) prior to my first triathlon.

When the day of the triathlon arrived, I thought I was ready but I panicked in the water during the swim segment and had to be pulled out by a lifeguard on one of the canoe boats that was there to make sure no one drowned. Although I was automatically disqualified, I competed in the cycling and the running portions since I was already there and I had trained for them. I felt both awful and excited at the same time. My head was saying, *I will never do another one of those crazy races again*, but my inner athlete was telling me, *You did pretty well finishing the bike and run; you just need to work more on your swimming. It's OK; you're still learning.* My inner athlete won out, and I trained over the winter for my next race the following spring. I finished the swim with no lifeguard assistance, and then competed in the bike leg. Embarrassingly, during my transition from the cycling leg to the running segment, I inadvertently began my run while I was still wearing my bicycle helmet. If my wife hadn't yelled for me to take it off, I probably would have worn it the entire three-mile run, but I managed to cross the finish line without being disqualified. I realized then that my Ageless Athlete journey had begun, all from a single thought. If it worked for me, it can work for you.

Triathlons may not be your passion or the direction you want to go, but think about an athletic activity you would really like to do or do better. Let your mind and imagination play. Your activity doesn't have to be something totally new or unfamiliar to you, but it can be. It can also be something you did earlier in life, something you currently do but not to your satisfaction, or something you always wanted to do. In any case, sit down in a quiet place, close your eyes, and see yourself engaging in your chosen athletic activity. Maybe you see yourself swinging a golf club and hitting the ball off the tee, straight down the middle of the fairway. Or you see yourself hitting the game-winning tennis ball into the corner of your opponent's court. Perhaps you're skating around an ice rink, controlling a hockey puck, and then slamming it into the goal. Maybe you're simply figure skating forward, or even backward, around a rink in a fluid motion with body poised and arms extended. Perhaps it's bowling a 200 game, pitching a horseshoe for a ringer, or making the perfect jump shot with the basketball going *swoosh* — nothing but net. What about hitting a home run and circling the bases? All of these can be athletic passions. The point is *you need something athletic to look forward to doing and getting better at it. This is your athletic passion.*

Your passion need not be a competitive activity against others. You might see yourself hiking to glorious mountain heights you never thought possible and in exotic places. You might simply try hiking around a beautiful lake in your own town, or becoming a hunter. I know a 60-year-old rifleman who climbs over logs and up a hill in his back yard to prepare himself for his trips to Alaska to hunt rare game. You might even see yourself deep sea fishing for sailfish, tuna, or bluefish, off a boat in the Caribbean. Such an athletic activity would require tremendous stamina since you could be holding a pole for hours on end while a several-hundred-pound fish fights to break the line. Fly fishing can teach you how to cast more accurately and give you more stamina and control for the day you reel in the big one!

Picture yourself doing your chosen activity in as much detail as you can. See yourself doing it well with coordination and accuracy. Envision how you feel engaging in your athletic activity. Experience the excitement; the adrenaline rush; the feeling of accomplishment; the thrill of success; and the pleasure of telling your family, friends, and fans what it's like to be athletic.

What about those of you who are already exercising on a treadmill, stationary cycle, or stairclimber at a local Y or health club...and hating almost every tedious minute of it? You need a passion, too, a goal that excites you. Did you know that race walking is a sport? So is stair racing — the Empire State Building has a famous stair race every year. And, of course, there are short and long running events, organized charitable walks, and bike rides to consider. A community where I lived, for example, sponsors an annual summer bike ride to raise funds for cancer survivor facilities and programs. It caters to all levels of athletes who ride anywhere from 25 to 100 miles and is called "The Connecticut Challenge" and many cancer survivors participate. The local press takes pictures of the riders at the start, the police stop traffic at every major intersection during the ride, athletes eat at numerous food stops along the way, and finishers have a big barbeque at the end.

Those of us with materialistic leanings can buy cool equipment, clothing, and other gear for our athletic activities. My latest "toy" is an Italian carbon fiber racing bike with aerodynamic carbon fiber wheels and a wireless computer with GPS that measures my distance, speed, elapsed time, and pedal cadence — all showing simultaneously on a tiny screen mounted on my handlebar. That really excites my Ageless Athlete and even makes him want to train even harder! After all, he is a triathlete and deserves the best I can give him.

So, let your imagination play! Picture yourself as an athlete. What do you see?

As you probably realize by now, training begins in the mind to think athletically. It is more than the power of positive thinking. It is internally teaching the nerve paths how to stimulate the muscles for a chosen athletic activity. Even as we picture ourselves in our chosen athletic activities, our brains are sending messages to our nerves and muscles about what they will need to learn, and we are creating positive images for our minds. You may need to do this mind training exercise several different times to see your athletic self fully, but you will see it if you keep up the training.

This little mind training exercise is called visualization, and you should use it throughout your training. Right now, at the beginning, I cannot stress enough the importance of letting your mind visualize your Ageless Athlete before you do any physical training. This is your core focal point or, as the Chinese say, your "chi" — where your athletic energy resides.

I can remember sitting in my office one day after I had given up smoking and had run the 5K race I described in Chapter One. This was years before I became a triathlete and I was asking myself if this running thing was merely a passing fancy I would get bored with and let go over time, or whether I was really interested in competing in more races. After all, I had never acted like an athlete before and had a difficult time believing the fun and excitement would continue. So did I like what it did for me enough to keep it up indefinitely?

My answer was a cautious yes because I hadn't been running for very long, so I worried I was reacting to a short-term runner's high. Running made me feel like an athlete and that was very new to me. But somehow, deep inside me, it seemed natural, like a part of my being, and I started to realize its absence from most of my life made me feel incomplete and unhappy. The thought that I could be an athlete for the rest of my life actually brought tears to my eyes. I was in touch with a part of me that could give me great joy and comfort. I was communicating with my Ageless Athlete and, although I didn't know it at the time, I was adding a major new dimension to who I was and how I lived my life. I had a deep feeling of calmness and excitement at the same time, like my life now had a meaningful purpose, and a purposeful meaning. I was awakening an element of my being I hadn't been aware of before. I was feeling more whole.

Before that day of questioning in my office, I didn't understand how exercising my body in a positive, purposeful way could change my mental outlook. That's what I want you to feel — and you can. Your Ageless Athlete is an inner part of you that you've previously neglected, perhaps out of ignorance, perhaps out of forgetfulness. The reason doesn't matter now, however, because you and your Ageless Athlete have been re-united or, as it was for me, perhaps this is your first introduction.

When you choose your athletic activity to visualize, first, choose one that involves some major muscle groups beyond pushing the buttons on a TV remote or the keys on a computer keyboard. Get your whole body, including your heart, into action. Your heart is a muscle that pumps blood throughout your body, so it needs strengthening. The blood from your heart then carries oxygen to your other muscles so they can continually function. So the stronger your heart is, the more oxygen it can pump to your other muscles, and the stronger and more responsive they will be.

Second, make sure your athletic activity will allow you to keep improving your strength, speed, endurance, technique, skill, or a combination of any of these. As you continually train, you should not only be getting more physically fit, but you should also be developing an increased ability and skill to perform more effectively at your chosen athletic activity. That's one of the big differences between exercising and training. When you exercise, your goal is generally to get fitter or thinner, to reduce body fat, or to develop more muscle definition without having any real athletic goal or passion. Training not only takes into account all these generic elements, but it also adds the specific needs and goals of your athletic activity to them — an athletic activity you have chosen to be passionate about.

In running a race, for example, the thinner you become (while developing your leg and upper body muscle strength), the less weight you have to carry on the run, and the faster and more mobile you become. All this increases your speed and ability to go further with the same amount of energy output. But if, for example, your arms are flailing about or going across your body instead of back and forth parallel to your body in the same direction you are running, you'll certainly be exercising but you'll be wasting energy that could be translated into more speed and endurance. Similarly, in swimming, the more you swim the stronger your shoulder and back muscles will get (and leg muscles if you remember to kick), which should enable you to go faster and farther in the water. If, however, you don't keep your body straight and learn proper stroke mechanics, again you'll be exercising and getting fitter, but the energy the added strength provides will be dissipated in useless exertions not related to improving your ability at the sport. Just compare Olympic swimmers to beginning swimmers. The beginners are splashing and twisting their bodies in various lateral directions, but for all their effort, are hardly advancing forward in the water. Olympic swimmers' strokes, on the other hand, are smooth and quiet, their bodies are moving along as straight as an arrow, and they are scary fast. Obviously, conditioning is a major factor in speed, but without proper technique, a large part of that conditioning goes to waste.

Third, choose an athletic activity you can train for before or after work and on weekends without a lot of travel or other hassles. Finally, and most important, choose something that will make you proud, that you can share (and boast about) with others. After all, your Ageless Athlete needs recognition for his or her accomplishments!

To sum up, unlike mere exercise endeavors, being an athlete helps focus and channel your motivation so you will train better and be able to achieve each goal you set so you can move on to the next one.

CHAPTER FIVE — SOME BASIC TRAINING PRINCIPLES

The previous chapter was aimed at awakening your Ageless Athlete, choosing an athletic activity, and making sure it is something you can and want to do. Although it is beyond the scope of this little book to discuss specific training programs for all the different athletic activities and training levels, there are some basic training principles I would like to pass on. I assume most of you probably haven't exercised much before reading this book. On that basis, this chapter will discuss some general training principles that I follow, which should apply to any athletic activity. The next chapter will discuss some specific training activities you can implement as a core program for whatever athletic endeavor your Ageless Athlete wishes to pursue.

Before you start training your Ageless Athlete, it is critical that you know your physical condition. Get a physical if you haven't had one recently. Training puts stress on the body and, as any properly trained athlete knows, you must know what your body can handle. This begins with letting a doctor examine your physical condition. I actually took a stress test before I started running. Also, if you experience any acute pain or injury during your training, see a doctor right away so you don't make it worse and can find out how to get back on track.

The Three Key Principles

When I went back to graduate school to study exercise physiology (another adventure my Ageless Athlete led me on), I learned that all training is based on two main principles: *repetition* and *progressively increasing resistance or difficulty level,* with a third interwoven principle called *specificity of training.* These three work together as you train. If you're a tennis player working on developing your serve, for example, begin your training by throwing the ball in the air, trying to give it the correct height and projection repeatedly until it is consistently correct. That's the *repetition* element. Then add bringing your racket into position as you throw the ball in the air. This is the *increased difficulty* element since you now have both arms involved at the same time, so you must stabilize your body to handle the arm activities. Next, *repeat* the ball throwing with this additional racket element until it is consistently correct and then add hitting the ball as it comes down — a *further difficulty* level. Keep doing this until it becomes fast, accurate, and consistent enough to produce a good serve. Then add more difficulty by trying to hit the ball at certain spots on the other side of the net and adding the spin. Get the picture?

The *specificity of training* element comes from what you're doing as it relates to your chosen athletic activity. In the tennis serve example, the training you're doing is exactly what you'll need to do in competition — it is specific to your sport of tennis. The more specific the training is to your chosen activity, the more effective it will be since you're actually strengthening and training your muscles in the exact way you want them to perform.

If you're training for a 5K (3.1 mile) race, begin by running a short distance that you can handle — say, a half mile — three, four, then five times per week for a few weeks until it becomes comfortable to you (*repetition*). Do the run in the middle of a mile-and-a-half walk (walk a half mile, run a half mile, then walk the final half mile). Then *increase the difficulty* by adding, say, another half mile to one of the weekly walk/runs, and extend the total walk/run to two or two-and-a-half miles (walk, run, walk, run, walk). Then add that second half-mile run to additional weekly walk/runs until all your walk/runs include two half miles (or a total of one full mile) of running. Then gradually shorten the walk time between the runs and add additional half miles until you're comfortably doing four miles of running with no walk intervals.

This process of going from half-mile run intervals to four-mile steady runs several times per week will probably take a couple of months to accomplish because, as a rule of thumb, do not increase your weekly run total by more than 10 percent per week. Next add in resistance (another way to *increase difficulty*) by adding some hills into the run and by running speed intervals (short periods of time or distance during the run where you run faster). The hills and intervals should initially only be included in one or two (and not on consecutive days) of your weekly runs because your body will need recovery time to adapt to this increased resistance and difficulty. Once this becomes comfortable, add more hills to increase your strength and power and more distance to the speed intervals. That's the *progressive increase in difficulty* element that will produce increasingly faster runs since the speed intervals will get longer and longer until the entire run is at the interval speed. That's how you become a faster runner. And, as with the tennis serve example, since you're actually running as you do the repetitions and increased difficulty, you're training your muscles to be stronger in the exact way you'll need to run the 5K race. This is the *specificity of training* principle.

The physiological underpinning of these three training principles is *muscular and neurological learning and adaptation*. The muscles become stronger from the increased stress on them, caused by the repetition and increases in difficulty, which helps them become more able to bear further increased resistance and difficulty levels. And since your brain sends electrical signals through nerves to your muscles to tell them how to act, the repetition, coupled with the specificity, teaches both the muscles and nerve connections how to do the given training element more efficiently and effectively. In our tennis serve example, coordination and accuracy improve as the hand and arm muscles learn the motions involved, and the muscles get stronger from practicing the elements so that, as time goes on, racket speed increases, resulting in a faster serve and better placement (where you want the ball to land). In the running example, adding distance to the runs increases the heart's ability to pump oxygen to the body more efficiently, resulting in less fatigue, and the slow-twitch muscles (that give endurance) also become stronger, resulting in longer endurance and less risk of injury. The hill and speed work also increase muscle strength, particularly the fast-twitch muscles (that give speed and power), so that you keep getting faster. And again, since you're doing what you will be doing in the race, namely running, the specificity is as good as it gets.

Later I'll discuss core strength training programs, which won't involve as much specificity. While specificity is very important in training, the body's ability to handle the specific athletic training requires a core level of strength and endurance to build from. You wouldn't put a 15-pound bowling ball in a young child's hand, for example, unless she or he is the child of Arnold Schwarzenegger. The child wouldn't even be able to lift the ball let alone throw it straight down a bowling lane, and would no doubt get hurt trying. Instead, you would start the child with a ball that weighs eight pounds or less and increase the weight of the ball as he or she gets stronger. But to get stronger, the child needs to develop some core muscle strength, which is not directly related to throwing a bowling ball.

I hope these examples give you a basic idea of how the body reacts to training. I will now make a **bold** statement I want you always to remember: ***Strength increases occur during recovery, not during the training activity itself.*** In fact, lack of recovery time leads to injury. While we're engaged in our training activity, we're actually tearing down our muscles because of the repetition and resistance. Then, during our recovery days (our days off from training), the muscles are not only able to rebuild what has been torn down, but they also add more muscle to better handle the next time they have to train and even do more.

Our Marvelous Bodies

The body is an amazingly adaptive organism. Since this adaptation is progressive, the more we train, with proper recovery intervals, the stronger we get and the more skilled we become at doing whatever it is we are training for. This happens regardless of age and training level when we start. Even if you can hardly climb a staircase, if you train at it, you will get stronger and better able to do it.

Before going further, I want you to picture your body. Picture your skeleton with all the bones that connect to each other, most of them through joints. Get a picture of the body's skeleton from your old biology book, an encyclopedia, or the internet. Look at how all the bones fit together. The hand connects to the lower arm at the wrist joint. The lower arm connects to the upper arm at the elbow joint. The upper arm connects to the shoulder and the back at the shoulder joint. The hip acts as a center joint between the spine (which supports the upper body) and the legs. The thigh bone connects to the hip and, through the knee joint, the lower leg connects to the thigh bone. Finally, of course, the foot connects to the lower leg through the ankle joint. As you can see, there are many interconnected movable bone parts.

Now, think of how all these bones actually connect and move. Yes, it is through the muscles. Muscles attached to all our bones keep them in place and extend across the joints to enable them to move. Simply bending your forearm, for example, recruits muscles that attach to the front of your upper arm bone and extend across your elbow joint to the front of your lower arm bones. You also have muscles that attach in the back of your upper arm bones and go across the elbows to the back of the lower arm bones. Bending your forearm contracts the muscles in front (biceps) and relaxes the muscles in the back of your arm (triceps). Straightening your forearm contracts the triceps in the back of your arm and relaxes the front bicep muscles. That's how we move. Every bend and extension of a body part involves some muscle contracting and an opposite one relaxing. Every time you make any movement, you're using muscles in that way. Amazing, isn't it? What a magnificent specimen of nature the human body is!

OK, so now you see that muscles control movement of the bones, and bone movement is how we do things. You need the bones in your fingers to grasp a ball, and the muscles in your fingers move the finger bones in the proper way to hold the ball. The reason we can stand upright is because the muscles on both sides of our legs keep the leg bones straight, while the hip bone, in turn, holds up the upper leg bone using muscles that attach to both. At the same time, the muscles from the spine run down your back and attach to the hip bone so the spine can stay up and straight, and even the head stays upright because the neck muscles attach to the skull and shoulder bones to keep the neck bones straight.

The stronger your muscles are, the better they will be able to do their jobs and take on other activities, as well. Let's go back to the tennis serve illustration. When your arm throws the ball in the air and your racket is back for the swing, your core body needs to remain straight and balanced and your legs need to be properly positioned. Then when your arm brings the racket forward to hit the ball, you won't lose your balance, wobble, or move in a way that throws your arm out of position. This means your body muscles must be strong enough to keep you properly aligned. So the serve actually involves your entire body, not just your arms. So, simply building your arm muscles without also building your core and leg muscles will not be enough training to engage in the athletic of tennis because as your arms get stronger and you swing that racket harder, your arm momentum will increase and pull your body around unless your legs and core muscles are strong enough to maintain their proper positions.

The point is, you can't simple aim your training at the specific muscles involved in your actual athletic activity. You must aim it at the entire body because, in reality, your whole body is involved in whatever you do. So you need a balanced training program for the whole body that involves the underlying principles of, you guessed it, repetition and increased difficulty/resistance with specificity interwoven into the process.

CHAPTER SIX — DEVELOPING A TRAINING PROGRAM

Now that you're all psyched and ready to go, aim your Ageless Athlete in the right training direction. Aerobic training and strength training are essential ingredients to success for all athletic activities, in addition to your specific training for your chosen athletic passion.

Playing tennis for an hour requires a certain amount of stamina. This comes from training your heart and muscles to endure the hour of running around the court and hitting the ball hard with your racket. Walking an 18-hole golf course (even in flat Florida) while swinging a golf club between 80 and 120 times (depending on your skill level) also requires several hours of endurance. Bowling several games in succession also requires stamina and strength so that you don't fatigue and lose your accuracy or, worse yet, throw your arm or back out. Or, how about mountain climbing? I can't think of a sport that requires more aerobic capacity both to climb up against gravity, and to handle the decreased level of oxygen in the air as the climber ascends to the higher altitudes. Without muscle development, particularly in the legs, meeting the challenges presented by such obstacles as steep inclines, rocks, and roots would prove difficult.

Many exercise enthusiasts, often called "gym rats," spend hours hanging around fitness clubs, doing both aerobic and strength training just for the sake of fitness.

If that's sufficient motivation, then more power to them. But I use aerobic training and weight training to assist me in becoming better at my chosen sport. They are part of being an athlete. Since my Ageless Athlete participates in triathlons (an endurance sport), my aerobic training is more specifically geared to bike rides and runs that simulate what I'll be doing in a race. That would not be the case, however, for a tennis player whose stamina requirements for his or her tennis matches come from a more general aerobic training process.

Conversely, my strength training is more general and somewhat limited since it's aimed at giving the muscles I use in a triathlon more strength to swim, bike harder, and run faster. A weight lifter would have an entirely different and more intense weight training program. The point is, there are two sets of training elements in any sport or other athletic activity: *the general* and *the specific* and they will often vary depending on the athletic activity.

So, by now, you are probably asking, "Why is he telling me all this, and how does it relate to my Ageless Athlete and his or her training?" The answer is simple. I want you, as an Ageless Athlete, to understand why certain training elements are an integral part of getting better at your chosen athletic activity, even though they may not even seem related to it. Think of Tiger Woods, perhaps the best golfer of all time. Did you know a major part of his training involves weights and running? The effects can be seen in how far he can drive a golf ball down the fairway and in how strong and unfatigued he still remains by the 18th hole of the fourth round of a tournament when he is either extending his lead or coming from behind for a victory. Serena Williams, one of the greatest ever women tennis players, also works with weights and does aerobic training and it shows in how hard she can hit a winner and how fast she can cover the court even in the third set after two hours of a difficult tennis match. Both general aerobic and strength training, as well as the specific training in your chosen athletic activity, are key elements in a balanced training program.

Aerobic Training

Since, as you already know from the last chapter, training involves repetition and progression, you need to train on a consistent recurrent basis, with sufficient recovery time between training sessions. Getting the aerobic base that will improve your stamina means starting with at least three aerobic training sessions per week, then building to four or more, depending on your athletic activity and how much time you have available, considering you need to train at your specific sport as well as live the rest of your daily life. The purpose of each aerobic session is to elevate your heart rate to increasingly higher levels without becoming anaerobic (out of breath). When you reach an anaerobic state, your muscles cease being able to absorb sufficient oxygen from your blood stream and start to shut down because of lactic acid buildup. This will lead to a "bonk" where you must either slow down, stop, or even be unable to continue the activity.

For most, the tools for aerobic training are the legs. Since your legs contain your largest groups of muscles, their need for oxygen, which is at the heart (no pun intended) of their ability to engage in aerobic training, is great. Increasing their activity level will stimulate your heart to pump more oxygen to the muscles in your legs. This in turn will give you more endurance and stamina, as you repeat and progress in your aerobic training, by strengthening your heart muscles and by increasing your leg muscles' capacity to absorb and utilize the oxygen being pumped. As you get better at your chosen athletic passion, the repetition and progressive time increases in the aerobic training make the leg muscles stronger and more efficient and you become faster and can go further. The legs are not the only tools for aerobic training, however. Rowing and swimming are also excellent upper body exercises that build aerobic capacity and stamina.

Whether you're training indoors on a treadmill, elliptical, stairmaster, stationary cycle, Nordic track, or rowing machine, or whether you're outdoors walking, running, cycling, inline skating, cross country skiing, swimming, or rowing a boat, you need to achieve a certain sustained effort level to make your activity aerobic. To put it simply, your effort level should be enough to work your heart muscle, but you should still be able to speak short sentences or phrases while you're doing it. Speak a few words; then take a breath. Repeat. To get to your optimum effort level, begin your aerobic activity slowly as a warm up (maybe 5 to 10 minutes), gradually increasing your effort until you break a sweat. At that point, you're at a good aerobic pace. Try to keep that pace for up to 20 minutes before slowing down and stopping. If you can't get to 20 minutes, do what you can and work up to 20 minutes over time. Try to make your total aerobic training session, including warm up and cool down, last at least a half hour.

After a few weeks, or possibly even a few months, you will probably find that your half hour of aerobic training will increase to as much as an hour. That's cooking! Again, the key is to do it consistently — at least three times per week. Lengthen the aerobic portion of your training sessions a few minutes per session each week, but add no more than 10 percent to your prior week's total. If the aerobic portion of each of your workouts is 20 minutes, for example, and you do that three times per week, you have 60 minutes of aerobic training for the week. The next week you can increase your aerobic training to 66 minutes by adding two minutes to each of the three aerobic portions of your workouts or by adding three minutes to two of the three workouts. This type of progressive increase in aerobic training lessens the risk of injury as well as the buildup of fatigue, which can have a cumulative effect on you as the weeks progress.

Increasing the amount of your aerobic training each week will cause your body to adapt to your level of aerobic effort (your pace) and the time you spend at it, and you'll increase both just to get to your sweat level. That means you're getting fitter. This aerobic training should always remain part of your training regimen. You'll be adding strength training and specific athletic training to it, not in place of it.

Strength Training

Strength training is essentially using weight or other resistance against the muscles as you're contracting them for a particular movement. You can even use your own body weight and the forces of gravity. You do this all the time in your daily life. Carrying the shopping bags from the supermarket to your car contracts muscles in your arms, back, and chest to hold the weight of the bags. Lifting or pushing a couch out of the way to vacuum involves using your muscles against the resistance of the couch. Even the back-and-forth motion of moving the vacuum cleaner across the rug (assuming it's an upright vacuum) involves your arm and back muscles working against the resistance created by both the weight of the vacuum and the friction of it rubbing on the carpet. How about taking out the garbage or bringing a full laundry basket upstairs? Mowing the lawn, moving rocks, digging holes to plant bushes, and other yard maintenance and landscaping activities involve muscle movement against resistance. Shoveling snow can be even more demanding on the muscles, particularly with heavy wet snow where your arms, back, chest, and legs are all enlisted to do the shoveling. The harder the resistance, the more your muscles have to work.

The resistance actually tears down your muscles, which then rebuild on your non-strength training days and actually become stronger so they can better handle the resistance next time. This process of tearing down and rebuilding is how the muscles get stronger. The key is not to create too much resistance so that you damage your muscles and, equally important, the muscles need recovery days for the rebuilding and growth process.

Unfortunately, these daily activities are not enough to build the strength needed for most athletic activities. They are not sufficiently consistent or repetitious nor do they work the muscles enough to be of any real athletic benefit. This is where specific strength training comes in. It need not be complicated or require large expenditures on equipment. In fact, the following five strength training exercises use your body and gravity for resistance and yet are quite effective for general muscle development regardless of the athletic activity you choose:

Push ups. Lie on your stomach and lift your body up from the floor by extending your arms and keeping your body as straight as possible. This results in using your body weight and gravity as a resistance against extending your arms. This resistance acts on your triceps (the back of your upper arm) and your chest (pectoral) muscles, which are both contracting during the process and which, as a result, will strengthen through repetition. Your core body muscles (stomach, hips, and back) are also contracting to keep your body rigid while you push up from the floor. Repeat the push ups until your arms become fatigued enough that they can't lift your body anymore.

Sit ups. In a sit up, you contract your stomach muscles to pull your upper body toward your lower body. Lie face up on the floor with your legs bent at the knees and your arms crossed on your chest. Next, pull your upper body up toward your bent knees while keeping your legs and butt stationary. The weight of your upper body, together with gravity, creates the resistance. Repeat the sit ups until your muscles fatigue (ache a little) and you can't lift your upper body anymore. Crunches are a variation on the sit up and involve less movement. Instead of lifting your entire upper body up from the floor, place your arms behind your head and just lift your shoulders off the floor and bend toward your legs. Don't lift your whole torso, just the upper part. Crunches are just as effective as full sit ups and put less strain on your back, although it usually takes a few more of them to reach your fatigue level.

Pull ups. Pull ups (sometimes called chin ups) require using a stationary bar mounted at a convenient place in your home, such as inside a door frame, at arms' length above your head. Grasp the bar while lifting your feet so that you are hanging in mid-air. Then pull yourself up using your arms to the point where your head and chin are above the bar level. This involves contracting your biceps and back muscles and, again, your body weight and gravity provide the resistance. If you can't do one of these the first time you try it (as I couldn't), simply lower the bar so you can lie on the floor under it and extend your arms up to grasp it. Then pull yourself up to the bar. As you get stronger, gradually increase the height of the bar. Repeat the exercise until your arms fatigue.

Squats: This simple exercise is excellent for working the front and back upper leg (hamstrings and quadriceps) and butt (gluteus) muscles. Stand against a wall with your feet about 12 inches apart. Bring your feet out in front of you, about 12 inches from the wall. Bend your knees and squat down (with your back still against the wall), so the lower part of your leg is vertical to the ground over your heel. Do not squat below the point where your upper and lower leg form a 90-degree angle at the knee, and do not let your knee extend further forward than the middle of your foot. Your legs should be at a right angle, and your butt should not go below the height of your knees. Squat down and then raise back up to standing position with your back always against the wall and your feet extended out from the wall at all times. Or, put an exercise ball (a rubber inflated ball six to 12 inches round) between the wall and your lower back (the small of your back). Extend your feet out further from the wall so that you keep the 90-degree angle. Repeat the up and down squat until your upper legs fatigue.

Calf raises. By far, this is the simplest exercise to do, but it only works the calf muscles in the lower leg. Using a staircase, stand on one step with your hand on the rail for balance. Then slide your feet back until just your toes and the ball of each foot remain on the step. Drop your heels below the height of the step and then bring them back parallel to the step. Repeat until your calves fatigue.

These five strength training exercises are effective ways to build and maintain upper and lower body and core strength without using any outside resistance. The next factors to consider are *how often* and *how much* you should do strength training.

How often. Generally speaking, it's not necessary to do strength training more than twice a week. You could build up to what I consider an ideal maximum of three times per week, but staying at two times per week is absolutely fine and effective (unless you want to be a body builder or weight lifter, which I assume is not the case). Since the strength training is meant to be added to your specific training for your athletic activity, don't do so much that you are too tired or too sore to do your athletic training. Each strength training session should be no longer than a half hour and, initially, even less as you gradually build up your strength. At least two to three days of recovery between sessions is important, particularly in the first couple of months, to allow your muscles to rebuild. After the second month, reduce your number of recovery days to no less than one between each strength training session but, again, do no more than three sessions per week. This means you will have two days off between sessions at least once per week.

How much. How much refers to three factors: the muscle groups worked, the number of repetitions performed, and the amount of resistance used. I like to work all the major muscle groups on a balanced basis — that is, work a muscle group and then the opposing muscle group. Opposing muscle groups refers to the muscles on opposite sides of the bones and joints. As you contract one of these muscle groups, the opposite one relaxes and stretches. The biceps and triceps are opposing muscle groups, as are the chest and back, and quadriceps and hamstrings. Generally there is no need to strength train more than these six muscle groups unless your chosen athletic activity involves other specific muscles that will need to be strengthened (maybe the forearm and fingers in bowling). Add stomach muscle sit-ups or crunches to your program to develop your core body. Initially, do not spend more than 20 minutes on these seven basic strength training exercises.

Do two to three sets of each exercise and rest a minute between each set. A set refers to the number of repetitions you do before stopping. Begin with eight repetitions at a sufficient amount of resistance so the exercise becomes somewhat difficult by the last couple of repetitions in the first set. By the third set, you may only be able to do six or seven repetitions, but gradually build up to eight repetitions per set. Then, over the course of the next few weeks, add another repetition and gradually build up to 12 repetitions in each set. A little "muscle burn" in the final repetitions is OK, but don't strain so hard that you risk injury to your muscles or tendons. Once you can do 12 repetitions in all your sets for a particular muscle group, add some more resistance and start at eight again.

Don't let your ego tell you the more weight or resistance you use, the stronger and more competitive you are. Aside from risking injury, by adding more resistance than you can really handle for the muscle group you are working on, you will likely start engaging other muscles for leverage, and then you will not be training the intended muscles as effectively. As a personal trainer, this is one of the most common mistakes I observe. Here's an example:

The standing curl is an exercise intended to train the bicep muscles in your front upper arm. The correct way to do the standing curl is to keep your back straight with knees relaxed and feet slightly apart for balance. For weight, let's assume you are using a straight metal bar about three feet long, and about an inch round, so you can grasp the bar near the ends with both hands and hold it parallel to the floor in front of you, waist high, and with your elbows bent and tucked in against your sides. Keeping the elbows tucked in (so that they act like a lever), lift the bar up and toward your chest to contract your biceps muscles. If the bar weighs too much, you'll end up recruiting back muscles into the exercise by arching your back or moving your elbows away from your sides and decreasing the use of your biceps. While you'll still be training muscles, you won't be effectively and efficiently training the ones you want.

Training Equipment

A key element of strength training is convenience. If the equipment is not readily available, you're less likely to do the training with sufficient consistency to get the intended benefit. I use a weight training machine I've had for years that I keep in my garage, so I have to see it every time I go to my car, which helps deter me from practicing my long-cultivated principle of "out of sight, out of mind" on my strength training. I also can't make the excuse that I have to drive too far to get to the machine. I realize the expense of purchasing such a machine may be impractical for many or even most of you, but you can often find a used one for sale, which will reduce your cost.

Additionally, there are several other less expensive alternatives. Joining a local Y or other fitness club will provide you with a large selection of weight machines, free weights, and other training equipment. But even this may be beyond your budget or not convenient enough to get to. If you have to drive more than 10 minutes, it's probably too far away. The closer it is, the more likely you are to go. The further away it is, the more excuses you will make for not going.

Bands and Tubes

Bands and tubes are both cheap and convenient and allow you to do your strength training virtually anywhere. Even though these are two different tools, they work the same way and are relatively interchangeable. You can purchase them at any fitness store and in many department stores that have an athletics section. I use them regularly and am amazed at how effective they are for such an inexpensive investment.

Bands are flat strips made of latex or another stretchy rubbery material. Each is about four to six inches wide and about three feet long. Tubes are like flexible water hoses that also stretch. They, too, are about three feet in length. Both bands and tubes come in a variety of thicknesses for a range of light to heavy resistance levels. Most tubes come with plastic or rubber handles attached, which makes them easier to grasp since, unlike bands that you can wrap around your hands, tubes are bulkier and not conducive to wrapping. Some bands come with handles, as well, to allow you to get a firm grip when doing an exercise. Some bands and tubes also have built-in ankle and thigh straps, which you can tie or attach around something sturdy and immovable, like a heavy bedpost leg. Some band and tube kits even come with a travel bag and various door and bar attachments.

Basic bands and tubes can range from $10 for a small set to $80 for a larger set with handles and additional attachments. Some bands and tubes come with instructions on how to use them in various strength training exercises, but many do not and, in either case, it is probably worth your while to purchase a DVD of instructions and workouts. You can find them at the same place you bought your tubes and bands, or on the internet. Your local Y or fitness club may also offer weekly classes in using bands and tubes they have at the facility to perform a variety of workouts under an instructor's supervision.

Bands and tubes stretch as you contract the muscles you're working on, which creates resistance. The thicker the band or tube, the more difficult it is to stretch, and the more resistance you create. Let's say you want to work your bicep muscle. Tie the band around the bottom of your foot or to a heavy object on the floor, such as a heavy sofa or bed leg. Wrap the other end of the band around your hand (or grasp the handle if it is a tube) and, with your elbow tucked stationary at your side, move your hand and lower arm upward toward your shoulder. As you bend your lower arm, the band or tube will stretch. The further you go with the bend, the greater the stretch, and therefore the more the resistance. It's like stretching a rubber band. You can use it to work just about every major muscle group virtually anywhere.

A word of caution: When using bands and tubes, make sure they don't develop holes or rips that could lead breakage while you are doing an exercise. This can result in a nasty, if not injurious, snap in your face or another part of your body. Hold them up to a light and examine them, and replace damaged bands or tubes immediately. Also, when attaching one end of the band or tube to your foot or to an object, make sure it is securely fastened so that, again, it does not snap back at you.

Weight Machines

Weight training machines fall into two categories: combination and separate machines. Combination machines have separate sections (called stations), each of which is aimed at training a specific muscle group. Bowflex is a combination machine, although it uses metal bands instead of weights for resistance. The combination machine in my garage gives me the ability to work each major muscle group by moving from station to station around the machine. If you decide to buy one instead of joining a Y or fitness club, it has the added benefit of not taking up a large amount of space.

Separate weight machines are usually aligned in what is called a circuit so you can go from one machine to the next to work each muscle group. Each machine in the circuit is designed to isolate and train a specific group of muscles while limiting the use of other muscles during the exercise being performed.

Both combination and separate machines are easier and quicker to work with than free weights (barbells and dumbbells) you only have to change the placement of a pin in a weight stack to select the amount of weight you want to use.

Free Weights

Free weights consist of barbells and dumbbells. A barbell is a round metal bar, which is held in both hands, about an inch in diameter and three feet long with an equal amount of weight on each end. A dumbbell is a small barbell about ten inches long with weight on each end for use by one hand. Barbells and dumbbells are "free" to move in any direction, unlike a weight machine that only moves in the direction necessary to exercise the intended muscles. You will, however, need to control the movement of the barbell or dumbbell so that it goes in the correct direction. This works your core muscles to stabilize your body and help you maintain balance. Just be sure to do each exercise properly to sufficiently work the intended muscles and factor in extra time for completing your workout since you'll have to add and remove the weights.

Training Exercises

Before beginning any type of strength training, do some "light resistance" or aerobic exercises to warm up your muscles by increasing your heart rate and blood flow. This reduces your risk of cold muscle strain or injury. I recommend starting with the larger muscle groups and working toward the smaller ones so that, as fatigue sets in, it's easier to keep going and, again, there is less risk of injury. Start by doing 10 to 15 minutes on a stationary cycle just to get your heart pumping and work up a little sweat. That way, your muscles are really warm and ready to go. Then do some sit ups. Since the only resistance is your own upper body weight, sit ups strengthen the stomach while warming you up.

My weight training routine takes 20 to 30 minutes, depending on the number of sets I do. Peruse the many books and websites of weight and other strength training exercises where you can find a large selection of both pictures and videos. There are many different weight, band, and tube training exercises available for each muscle group. The key is to do some form of muscle training for these main muscle groups on a regular (consistent) basis.

Now that you understand the basics, start doing them. They will become the foundation on which your Ageless Athlete will build your training program. Even before you get into significant training in your chosen athletic activity, make your aerobic and strength training programs a part of your weekly routine. Do them enough so that if you skip a training day, you miss it and feel bad! That feeling will become a great motivator for making your Ageless Athlete stronger and fitter.

Whether you start your specific athletic training as you do your core training depends on your fitness level and the nature of your athletic activity. You may find you can fit it in right from the beginning. Perhaps you have been dabbling at it for years and now want to take it to the next level. If you've already been engaging in your chosen athletic endeavor, continue to include it as part of your training regimen and add in the strength training. If you plan to increase your resistance levels, first determine whether your fitness level is sufficient to handle the increase. If not, simply maintain at a lesser level while you build up your core fitness. If you haven't been engaging in your chosen athletic endeavor, defer embarking upon the specific training or do it in a limited way while you build up your core fitness. Gradually, as you start feeling fitter, add in more specific athletic training.

The fitness training in this chapter will give you a new platform to begin the increased specific training effort to achieve your goals. Again, maintain a balance between your core fitness training and your specific training, but make both part of your training program. Take a tennis lesson every week, for example, and practice it three times a week while you also do your general fitness training two or three times a week. Or bowl six games a week — two at a time on three different days. Break the specific training into several sessions each week to stimulate the muscle and nerve memory needed for improving. Remember, repetition and recovery.

The point is to add in enough specific training to see if your chosen athletic activity is something you'll enjoy doing or one that you want to take to a new level (since you'll be working harder at it) if you've already been doing it for some time. Give it a chance. Stay at it for at least a couple of weeks or, even better, a month (unless you reach a point where you absolutely, positively can't stand it and will scream if you have to go another day). Don't worry about how well you're doing at your chosen activity — focus on whether you like it and feel you can improve. If you find your choice was a mistake, don't get discouraged. Try something else. Even if you go through several different intended athletic passions over a period of months, you're still doing something healthy for yourself and your Ageless Athlete is narrowing down the field of choices. Remember, even an elite athlete like Michael Jordan tried playing baseball and discovered he was happier with (and better at) basketball. Something will click if you stay with it long enough.

After I started running, I worked my way from three-mile races to 26.2-mile marathons. Then I decided I didn't like running so many miles. I was running five or six days per week and doing long runs twice a week. I found myself becoming negative about the long run days and wanting to avoid them. So I switched to cycling to compete in bicycle races since I had very developed thigh muscles, which gave me a lot of pedal power. But I soon got bored with just doing cycling and even missed the running (at least the shorter runs).

Then triathlons attracted my Ageless Athlete's attention because they seemed to involve virtually all the major muscle groups: back, chest, and arm muscles to swim; thigh and gluteus (butt) muscles to cycle; and hamstring and calf muscles to run. Triathlons didn't have the tedious training involved with marathon running, and saying "I'm a triathlete" sounded really cool, especially now since it's an Olympic sport and much more recognized as a true sport. Like I said before, Ageless Athletes like recognition for what they do.

When I started, however, I didn't know how to swim and, to this day, the swim is my weakest event in the triathlon although I am far better than when I began. I started with swimming at the local Y indoor pool. I figured since my two children were competitive swimmers when they were young, swimming was probably in my genes, too. Wrong! They must have gotten it from their mother. I could barely swim the length of the pool and my arms and legs were flailing all over the place. I was terrified of sinking and I must have looked like I was drowning because one of the lifeguards, who was also a swim coach, offered to give me lessons for free. I took advantage of his moment of pity and grabbed at the opportunity like a drowning person clutches for a life buoy.

Several lessons later, and after many days of pool swimming and gradually extending my distance up to a half mile, I signed up for my first triathlon. It involved swimming in open water which I had tried, very close to shore, a few times prior to the race. On race day, I went in the water with a wave of about 100 swimmers. I was getting banged around in the midst of the other swimmers as we headed toward the first marker buoy. I got scared. It was much further out than I had practiced. Again I thought I would drown, and I started imagining there were strange fish in the water ready to bite my feet. My lungs started tightening and I was gasping for air. Another swimmer saw me struggling and helped me back to shore (and sacrificed his own race to do it). I was so depressed and demoralized that I was ready to throw in the proverbial towel and go back to just running. But, with the encouragement of my wife and other triathletes whom I had befriended, I gave it another shot. This time, my training included much more open water swimming (with other swimmers alongside me to rescue me if I needed it) and I gradually started overcoming my fear. In my next race attempt, I stayed at the back of the starting wave of swimmers so I would not get bumped around and I actually finished the half-mile swim, got through the bike leg, and completed the run. I was exhausted but exhilarated. I had finished my first triathlon! I was an Ageless tri-Athlete. As time went on and I participated in more races, I discovered the good swimmers are often lousy runners and the good runners often can't cycle fast. So the triathlon was an opportunity for my Ageless Athlete to be in the middle of the pack at all three sports and still be competitive. Who would have ever thought mediocrity would be an asset in triathlons? Actually my Ageless Athlete prefers to think of it as having a balanced ability in all three disciplines.

So, my experience illustrates two lessons. First, whatever athletic endeavor you choose, it need not be a lifelong marriage. I went from running to biking to triathlons before I finally settled in (for now). If your first or second choice becomes unappealing, there are plenty of other athletic activities to look into. I mentioned Michael Jordan going from star basketball player to not-so-hot baseball player and back to basketball — now that he is retired from basketball, he has become a pretty good golfer. The key is to listen to your Ageless Athlete, and don't give up — which is part of the second lesson.

Second, just because your chosen athletic activity, or parts of it, are new and you may not be good at them initially, don't get discouraged. Every athlete starts at the beginning — keep at it for a while and you'll get better. If you need help, get it. Lessons are nothing to be ashamed of. Learning proper technique and training regimens from the beginning is far more efficient and easier in the long run than unlearning improper technique later or becoming exhausted or injured from overexertion. This brings us to another lesson: DO NOT OVERTRAIN.

Kent's Story

Beware. This story does not have a happy ending. It's here to illustrate an important training point: athleticism is a growth process and overtraining causes injury.

Kent was a 40-year-old businessman and computer potato. During a routine physical, Kent's doctor told him he was overweight and had dangerously high cholesterol. So Kent went on a strict diet and started to lose weight. He also accepted that, in addition to proper diet, exercising aerobically was a key ingredient to better health and a healthy lifestyle. Using his computer research, he found studies showing aerobic exercise not only burns calories and makes the heart stronger, but it also increases the production of "good" HDL cholesterol in the body, which counteracts some of the negative effects of "bad" LDL cholesterol.

So off Kent went to the fitness equipment store. Over the next six months, using the Weight Watchers counting method, he lost 50 pounds and, through using his newly purchased treadmill and stationery cycle, he worked up to running three miles at a time. In the spring, he took all his new-found fitness outdoors and started cycling. He purchased a new, high-quality hybrid bicycle (which is essentially a road bike with wider tires). He started cycling several days a week in addition to running on the non-bike days. Eventually he could bike 35 miles over rolling hills to his father's house and back. Kent had become an athlete. So pleased was Kent with his improvement that he started talking about doing a 5K running race and a century (100 mile) bike ride in the fall.

Then calamity struck. Kent did not understand the cumulative effects of training too much and too often. He was biking or running almost every day without giving his body time to recover so his muscles could become strong enough to endure the increased training loads. The body doesn't get stronger from the training. It gets stronger from the recovery days when it can rebuild and adapt to the increased training. Without the recovery time, the muscles become overstressed and start deteriorating. There are signs along the way — aches, fatigue, slowness, irritability, and other messages the body gives. Kent ignored them because he thought he was doing so well that he wanted to improve even faster. He thought more training would do it for him.

One morning when Kent got out of bed and put his foot down, his knee wouldn't straighten and he couldn't walk. Such injuries are the body's way of saying "slow down" when all other messages are ignored. But Kent did the right thing next. He went to the doctor for an examination and advice. The doctor told Kent he had inflamed the muscles around his knee and couldn't run or bike for a month. Kent was disappointed and angry.

Unfortunately, once Kent's training routine was broken, he was in trouble. He felt as if his body had failed him and, during the time he couldn't train, old thoughts about his lack of athleticism crept back and he became depressed. He continued to eat as if he was still training at the same level and the weight started to come back. He started eating more for solace and resurrected his old sedentary habits to fill the time the training used to take. In that short month of recovering from his injury, Kent had returned to his old self. He started taking a drug to lower his cholesterol and saw no reason to do more. Kent's Ageless Athlete was forced into retirement.

Athletic endeavors, like all other worthwhile pursuits, must be kept in balance. Kent was hypnotized by the excitement he was experiencing in improving as an athlete and he ignored a cardinal rule of training: exercise days stress the body and rest days allow the body to recover and make itself stronger for the next exercise day. Because Kent failed to take the required rest days, he stressed his body even more each exercise day until he eventually became injured.

On a happier note, Kent's training efforts so impressed his father that he also commenced a weight loss and training program. His wife had already been exercising and now they could do it together. Hiking became their athletic activity and today they regularly take vacations that involve hiking up mountains and enjoying both the satisfaction of their accomplishments and some beautiful mountaintop views. Ageless Athletes at 70 years old!

Also, as you increase your specific training in your athletic activity, you may need to cut back on your basic fitness training if you can no longer fit both sets of training into your schedule, or if the physical exertion involved in doing both is hindering your athletics training. Strength training three times a week for all your basic muscle groups may no longer be necessary given the athletic activity you are pursuing. Since I do triathlon training, for example, I don't need to do strength training for my legs as often since the cycling and running are strength training exercises. Swimming, too, is strength training for the back and chest. As a result, during triathlon season I'll usually do strength training only twice a week (sometimes even once a week just to keep the muscles toned and still attuned to the strength training), with fewer leg, back, and chest sets with less weight since I don't want these muscle groups to be too tired to do the swim, bike, and run training I need to do for racing. Even elite athletes and other seriously competitive athletes cut back on their strength training levels during the height of their competitive season. In the off season, I will cut back my triathlon training and add back in more strength training. Your particular athletic endeavor may not be competitive or seasonal like mine, and you may have time to do both strength training and your athletic training, or maybe the strength training is a key element of your athletic training (like in bowling or tennis). In those cases, there is no reason to cut back as long as you maintain a proper amount of recovery in your schedule. Again overtraining leads to injury.

If you wish to read more about training in specific athletic activities, there are already stores and libraries full of books on specific training programs and proper training techniques. My purpose is to get your Ageless Athlete on a right course so you will find these books useful and effective.

CHAPTER SEVEN — INJURIES

It's an unfortunate fact of life that all athletes become more prone to injury as they age. Ligaments, tendons, and muscles become less resilient and bones become more brittle. The good news is that athletic training slows the process; however, there are important procedures for athletes to follow as we age.

Stretching is first and foremost. Stretching preserves range of motion so that inadvertent overextension or twisting the wrong way becomes less likely to cause serious tearing and pulls. Ideally, stretching should be incorporated into every workout. After a ten-minute, non-strenuous warm-up, the muscles are sufficiently heated enough to be stretched. Stretching before warming up increases the risk that the stretch itself can cause a pull on a cold muscle. With the warm-up, the muscles are more supple and the stretches are more effective. All major muscles groups can benefit from stretching. The goal is to stretch the muscle to the point where it starts feeling uncomfortable but not painful and hold the stretch for 20 seconds to allow the muscle to relax in the stretch position. Then take a 20-second break and do it again. Three to five times for each stretch is generally enough. Over time, your flexibility will increase and you will be able to stretch further than when you started. Stretching the muscles you will be using in your training will enable them to respond with less tightness and more flexibility, which translates into more speed and power. At the end of a training session, do similar stretches to relieve any tightness the training may have caused and to start the release of lactic acid buildup, which occurs from strenuous training.

Even with the best stretching preparation, however, injuries do occur and you must know how to deal with them both emotionally and physically. When I started training for my first marathon, I increased my mileage too rapidly and developed a pain in the bottom of my foot, which was particularly excruciating when I got up in the morning and lessened as the day progressed. Unfortunately, at first it didn't prevent me from running, although the next morning the pain was even more excruciating. I hadn't read any books about marathon training or about the types of injuries that can result from running, so I had no idea how to deal with the injury. Finally, since it wasn't going away and it started interfering with my running, I went to a foot doctor and he immediately diagnosed my problem as plantar fasciitis, a common injury to runners that comes from overuse or improper or worn running shoes. My doctor told me the only cure was total rest and that, once it healed, I could resume running at a modest level and build my speed and mileage back at a slow pace. I lost several weeks of training, but still had enough time to build to a sufficient level of fitness to complete the marathon (which was still more than three months away). What I gave up, however, was a potentially higher fitness level, which might have resulted in a faster or less-arduous marathon. And I would have avoided the depression and irritability that three weeks off from training caused me. Remember that mind/body connection discussed in Chapter Four. I train, not only to race, but also to relieve stress and maintain emotional balance.

The lesson I learned from my injury was twofold. First, I learned to educate myself about implementing a proper training program, including knowing about potential injuries, their symptoms, and causes. Second, I learned patience. Training is not an overnight process, and the body needs time to develop additional strength and protections to recover and grow from the stresses the training causes. The positive cumulative effect from training is that over time, we get faster, stronger, and more powerful, and the negative cumulative effect from overtraining is that over time, our body is tearing down, our muscles are becoming weaker, and we are heading toward injury. Fatigue, restlessness, joint and muscle tightness, irritability, and sleeplessness are all signs of overtraining. The insidious part is that, as the body weakens, we think we're not training enough and we increase our training levels instead of resting more. Our mind says "Work harder," and it drowns out the screams from our body saying "Slow down and let me rest!" At that point, our body has only one avenue left to stop us — injury.

Another type of injury is accidental injury. I have fallen off my bike four times in the past ten years. One time I slipped on some sand and hit my head so hard on the pavement that my helmet cracked and I had short-term memory loss for several hours. Without the helmet, I probably would have had permanent damage. Another time, I was showboating on the bike in the middle of a short triathlon, lost control, and fell over at about 20 miles per hour. Although I was at such a high endorphin level that I got back on the bike (I only had about a quarter mile to go) and completed the run, the road rash was so severe that I could only sleep in one position on my back for a week. I took second in my age group and probably could have won if I had been more careful. The next two falls also occurred during races and resulted from road hazards (pothole and speed bump). Both times, the seriousness of the injury kept me from continuing the race and required medical assistance for the bleeding. The second of these happened at a world championship triathlon in France and I was heading for a top 10 finish in my age group, so I was depressed for weeks. Luckily, none of my injuries has been serious enough to end my triathlon "career."

The biggest challenge I have faced, however, has come, not from overtraining or accident, but from my genetics and body-aging process. I developed a severe case of degenerative hip joint arthritis, which had progressed enough to prevent me from running and interfered with my ability to pedal my bike. I was forced to have hip replacement surgery. As a result, my long-distance running and long-course triathlon days are over. I can still do sprint triathlons, which involve no more than three-mile run segments, and I'll need to do much of my run training in water and on elliptic machines or I run the risk of prematurely wearing out my new hip. Initially this was a major setback for my Ageless Athlete, but then he realized that, being an athlete, other athletic endeavors remained available. The sprint triathlons will still allow me to do what I love while motivating me to engage in full-body training, which is the reason I started doing triathlons in the first place. I can also pedal in longer cycling races, which allow me to focus on the activity I love most, while giving me another sport to participate in! And, I would be remiss if I didn't tell you how fast I was able to recover from the surgery because I was in impeccable shape going in and I knew how much I could push on the physical therapy because it is just like training — only at a different level with a different goal.

This brings up an important point. Training properly teaches us the difference between "good" pain and "bad" pain. Good pain is the burning sensation in our muscles and feeling of reaching a limit that comes from pushing ourselves beyond previous boundaries. When we feel it, we endure it for a short time and then stop because we know our bodies will need to recover from the effort. We then give our bodies that recovery time and accept a level of stiffness and maybe some achiness. Bad pain, on the other hand, is a sharp or acute pain that stops us in our tracks and results in injury. It can actually start as a sharp twinge in a muscle that will knot up into acute pain if we continue. Because of my fitness training and experience, my body knows the difference and I can use that knowledge to train properly and avoid bad pain.

While some injuries can be avoided and perhaps others cannot, no Ageless Athlete worth his or her salt ever gives up. He or she just shifts focus and looks for solutions, even if they appear to be second best. I expect to be an Ageless Athlete until the very end and I love living as a result. Never give up. Draw inspiration from the Hoyts and all the physically challenged athletes around you. It is the journey, not the destination, that brings the happiness.

PART C

EATING RIGHT AND OTHER TIPS

CHAPTER EIGHT — TRAINING TO EAT

I don't believe in diets; I believe in properly balanced eating habits. Diets, by definition, have a starting point and an ending point (usually much further away than we want it to be), and all diets involve sacrifice. When the Buddhists first said that life is suffering, I'm sure they were all on diets. Balanced eating habits shouldn't involve sacrifice or suffering. We all hate diets and can't wait to achieve our desired weight loss so we can return to "normal" eating. Balanced eating habits involve eating "normal" all the time.

Let's get back to our Ageless Athlete's body for a moment. We already know athletes need muscle strength and endurance to perform effectively. But the muscles also need to be able to repair, grow, and work properly. Food is the fuel for both. It provides the materials the muscles use to rebuild and develop from training, and it provides the energy for the muscles to actually do the training. The harder an athlete trains, the more food he or she will need to replenish and repair his or her muscles and build better fitness. The nature of a particular food is identified by its content of three key elements: carbohydrates, fats, and protein. Energy comes principally from carbohydrates and, at lower exertion levels, from fats. Protein is what the muscles need to repair and build. They should never be used as a source of energy, however, because that could ultimately tear down the muscles instead of building them.

So the question becomes: where and how does an Ageless Athlete get the right mix of carbohydrates, fats, and protein to maximize both the training effort and proper muscle development? The answer is: from balanced eating habits, not from diets of one type of food to the exclusion of others, or with quantity limitations that would starve a bird.

Think of your body as a finely tuned vehicle (maybe a sexy sports car or, if you're a big person, a Porsche Cayenne SUV) and food is what keeps it running. If you deprive a vehicle of gas and oil, it will slow down, get out of tune, and eventually stop running. Depriving your body of the types or amounts of food it needs will have the same effects.

You are no doubt familiar with the food pyramid the government and many nutritionists promote as a balanced way to eat. A version of it, prepared by the Massachusetts Institute of Technology, is pictured below and covers the major food groups and the suggested portions of each that a person should be eating. But as Ageless Athletes, we need to understand how the body uses food to produce energy and build muscle and how much food it takes to do this.

Calories Out and Calories In

I use calories to measure how much I eat since energy is measured in calories used (or burned) by the body during an activity. Calories consumed are derived from the food we eat. Our bodies burn calories all the time. To determine how many calories you need to consume each day to support your body's internal operating system and your other energy needs, you need to know your basal metabolic rate (BMR). Simply put, BMR is the amount of calories your body burns each day just to keep you alive. This includes breathing in and out, keeping your heart pumping blood, digesting your food, maintaining your body's temperature, and all the other processes that go on in your body. In the average person (not an athlete), BMR can use up to about two-thirds of your total daily caloric intake.

Imagine yourself lying in bed all the time. This is only a hypothetical, so don't dwell on it too long. Your BMR is the amount of calories your body will burn while you're lying there for 24 hours. BMR does not take into account any physical activity you perform. Once you know your BMR, add in your level of physical activity and figure out how many calories you're burning each day. Then use this to determine how many calories you need to consume per day to lose, gain, or maintain your weight.

You can determine your BMR in a totally rested state using a basic formula and, unless you are extremely muscular or overweight, you will have a pretty accurate idea of the number of calories you need to consume daily just to keep your body working. Since muscles increase your metabolic rate, and fat can have a negative impact on your metabolic rate, BMR is affected by both of these. The most accurate way to measure the impact of these on your BMR is to have a body fat percentage analysis done. Then a special formula can be applied to determine your BMR. For most of you, this added body fat analysis step is probably not readily available, so just use a standard BMR formula (such as the Harris-Benedict formula), which takes into account weight, height, age, and gender. For the purposes of your training, it should serve as a reasonable starting point.

BMR Formula

For <u>men</u>:

BMR = 66 <u>plus</u> (your body weight in pounds multiplied by 6.2) <u>plus</u> (your height in inches multiplied by 12.7) <u>minus</u> (your age multiplied by 6.76)

For <u>women</u>:

BMR = 655 <u>plus</u> (your weight in pounds multiplied by 4.35) <u>plus</u> (your height in inches multiplied by 4.7) <u>minus</u> (your age multiplied by 4.7)

Of course, no one lies in bed all the time, right? So, even if you lead an inactive life, you will still be burning some additional calories; therefore, the standard for determining the inactive person's BMR is to multiply the results from the above formulas by 1.2. This increases to 1.375 for a mildly active person and can go as high as 1.9 for a highly active person.

If all this math is too complicated and you just want someone to give you a BMR number to work from, the following pages include charts based on the above formulas, to show BMRs for various heights (in feet and inches), weights (in pounds) and ages (in years), using the 1.375 multiplier. While the charts are not as accurate as using the formulas I've just discussed, you may still find them a useful starting point. The numbers in **bold** in the tables are the BMR for the height (on left) and weight (on top). Choose the BMR closest to your age, height, and weight and, for good measure, subtract 50 from the selected BMR (just to err on the side of fewer calories).

BMR Charts

Male -- Age: 40 yrs

Ht/Wt	150lbs	165lbs	180lbs	195lbs	210lbs	225lbs
5'7"	2168	2296	2424	2552	2680	2808
5'9"	2203	2331	2459	2587	2715	2843
5'11"	2238	2366	2494	2622	2750	2878
6'1"	2273	2401	2529	2657	2785	2913
6'3"	2308	2436	2564	2692	2820	2948

Male – Age: 50 yrs

Ht/Wt	150lbs	165lbs	180lbs	195lbs	210lbs	225lbs
5'7"	2075	2203	2331	2459	2587	2715
5'9"	2110	2238	2366	2494	2622	2750
5'11"	2145	2273	2401	2529	2657	2785
6'1"	2180	2308	2436	2564	2692	2820
6'3"	2215	2343	2471	2599	2727	2855

Male – Age: 60 yrs

Ht/Wt	150lbs	165lbs	180lbs	195lbs	210lbs	225lbs
5'7"	1982	2110	2238	2366	2494	2622
5'9"	2017	2145	2273	2401	2529	2657
5'11"	2052	2180	2308	2436	2564	2692
6'1"	2087	2215	2343	2471	2599	2727
6'3"	2122	2250	2378	2506	2634	2762

Male – Age: 70 yrs

Ht/Wt	150lbs	165lbs	180lbs	195lbs	210lbs	225lbs
5'7"	1889	2017	2145	2273	2401	2529
5'9"	1924	2052	2180	2308	2436	2564
5'11"	1959	2087	2215	2343	2471	2599
6'1"	1994	2122	2250	2378	2506	2634
6'3"	2029	2157	2285	2413	2541	2669

Female - Age: 40 yrs

Ht/Wt	100lbs	115lbs	130lbs	145lbs	160lbs	175lbs
5'0"	1628	1718	1808	1898	1988	2078
5'3"	1648	1738	1828	1918	2008	2098
5'6"	1668	1758	1848	1938	2028	2118
5'9"	1688	1778	1868	1958	2048	2138
6'0"	1708	1798	1888	1978	2068	2158

Female – Age: 50 yrs

Ht/Wt	100lbs	115lbs	130lbs	145lbs	160lbs	175lbs
5'0"	1563	1653	1743	1833	1923	2013
5'3"	1583	1673	1763	1853	1943	2033
5'6"	1603	1693	1783	1873	1963	2053
5'9"	1623	1713	1803	1893	1983	2073
6'0"	1643	1733	1823	2013	2003	2093

Female – Age: 60 yrs

Ht/Wt	100lbs	115lbs	130lbs	145lbs	160lbs	175lbs
5'0"	1498	1588	1678	1768	1858	1948
5'3"	1518	1608	1698	1788	1878	1968
5'6"	1538	1628	1718	1808	1898	1988
5'9"	1558	1648	1738	1828	1918	2008
6'0"	1578	1668	1758	1848	1938	2028

Female – Age: 70 yrs

Ht/Wt	100lbs	115lbs	130lbs	145lbs	160lbs	175lbs
5'0"	1433	1523	1613	1703	1793	1883
5'3"	1453	1543	1633	1723	1813	1903
5'6"	1473	1563	1653	1743	1833	1923
5'9"	1493	1583	1673	1763	1853	1943
6'0"	1513	1603	1693	1783	1873	1963

BMR tells you how many calories you need to eat each day to stay at your same weight with very limited exercise. If you eat more than that, you will likely gain weight and, if you eat less, you will likely lose weight. Also, if your Ageless Athlete starts adding the training we previously discussed to each day's schedule, the number of calories you burn each day will increase, which means you will need to eat more to stay at the same weight or, perhaps more importantly to many budding Ageless Athletes, by simply not eating more, you will lose weight. I don't know about you, but to me that certainly doesn't sound like dieting!

Let's take the case of a 45-year-old male, who is 5'9" and weighs 180 pounds (we'll call him "Lance"). Interpolating from the charts, we would give him a BMR of about 2,400 calories per day. Now let's say he starts briskly walking an additional three miles each day, six days per week, for a total of 18 miles each week. The average person (depending on weight) generally burns about 100 to 120 calories per mile walked, which would, assuming an average of 110 calories per mile, be 1,980 additional calories burned per week by Lance. If Lance eats only his 2,400 BMR calories each day, he will lose well over a half pound of weight each week simply from the additional walking since a pound is 3,500 calories and the additional 1,980 calories is more than half of that. If Lance adds in weight training three days per week for about a half hour each time, he will burn approximately 700 calories more each week and, if he drops his daily calorie intake by a mere 300 calories per day (which would still keep him well above his bed-resting BMR), he would lose almost a pound and a half per week. He would probably lose more because even after he finishes his training activity, his body will continue to burn calories at a higher rate for a period of time before settling back to its BMR rate. As Lance's Ageless Athlete gets more fit, he can increase both training amount and intensity and lose more pounds each week. Plus, since muscle increases metabolic rate, his added muscle development will result in a higher BMR. So, as he gets stronger, Lance will be burning more calories even while he is in an inactive state.

There you have it; you don't have to eat less to lose weight; you simply have to let your Ageless Athlete train and the pounds will come off automatically. You can speed up the process a little by cutting back on your daily calorie intake, but don't go below your BMR. Remember, your body needs the calories to continue operating and to create the energy necessary to train.

Now you have the basic weight control rule: *calories eaten must not exceed calories burned.* The Harris-Benedict BMR formula (and applying the 1.3 multiplier) should give you a reasonably accurate starting point for the number of calories you can eat each day to maintain your weight without adding in the training.

Following is a chart which I have created of some estimated average number of calories burned per hour for various common athletic activities. These are estimates only and will vary depending on a variety of factors such as weight, gender, speed, intensity, etc. Since we continue to burn calories at an accelerated rate for several hours after we stop exercising, I would add another 10 to 15 percent of calories to the calculations. Tape the chart to your refrigerator door. Then every time you open it, the chart will remind you how much effort it takes to burn the calories you're about to eat. Trust me; it's much easier to take the calories in than to burn them off.

Activity	Calories/hour
Aerobics:	400-500
Dancing:	300-400
Basketball:	450-600
Bowling:	150-200
Boxing:	400-550
X Country Skiing;	450-600
Cycling:	450-650
Downhill Skiing:	200-300
Football:	500-650
Golf:	200-250
Hiking:	350-450
Ice Hockey:	500-650
Horseback riding;	175-200
Ice Skating:	350-450
Kick boxing:	450-600
Paddleball:	500-650
Roller Skating:	500-650
Rowing machine:	450-650
Running:	600-800
Ski machine:	350-450
Soccer:	600-800
Squash:	700-900
Swimming:	600-800
Tennis:	450-600
Walking:	250-450
Water Skiing:	450-550
Weight lifting:	300-450

Healthy Eating, Healthy Food

Calories consumed and burned are not the whole eating story, however. What you eat is at least as important, and probably more important, than how many calories you eat. Let's look at the USDA food pyramid of suggested types of foods and portions that make up a healthy eating program:

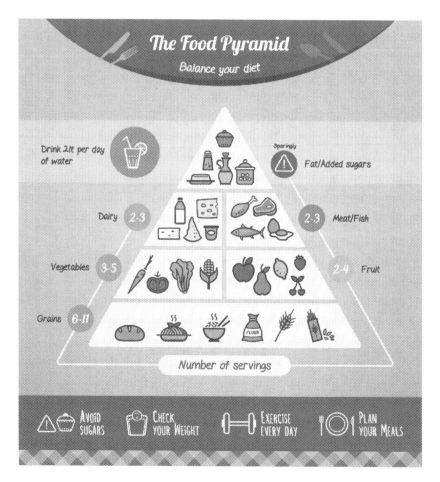

Tufts University has added eight 8-ounce glasses of water to the pyramid for people over 70 years of age, but this should apply to all adults. Although water is not technically a food, it is absolutely necessary for your body to function properly. Water flushes our digestive systems and keeps us properly hydrated, the latter being extremely important for Ageless Athletes since sweating from training will remove water (as well as needed sodium and potassium) from the body. I drink Propel or G-2 (by Gatorade) when I train and, on hotter days, I add in sodium/potassium tablets for longer training sessions.

Drink a pint (16 ounces) of water per hour starting about 20 minutes into your training and then at 10 to 15 minute intervals through the balance of your training time. If you get thirsty, your body has lost too much water, which means your blood is thickening. That makes it more difficult for your heart to pump, and this causes your heart rate to increase significantly. This in turn means less oxygen is getting to your muscles and you will become anaerobic (or worse, overheated and dangerously dehydrated), which will quickly end your training session. So if you get thirsty, take a water break to allow your body to come back to an aerobic state before resuming your training.

During your training, drink to avoid becoming thirsty. Also, drink water throughout the day to keep your system flushed and your body properly hydrated. You're properly hydrating if your urine is virtually clear to light yellow. If it is a bright or concentrated yellow, you're not drinking enough water. And don't be surprised if your frequency of urination increases. That's not a bad thing.

Back to what you eat. I use the food pyramid as my basic guideline to eating while I train; however, I tend to eat less of the bread, pasta, cereal, and rice group and more of the vegetable group than the pyramid suggests since there are more nutrients in the vegetable group and they have a sufficient carbohydrate count for my training activities. Raw vegetables and fruits are the most nutritious since cooking destroys a large quantity of their nutrients. So a salad with raw broccoli, beets, mushrooms, cauliflower, peppers, and some grilled chicken is a great meal for me and, with some low-calorie Caesar dressing, it is absolutely delicious and filling.

While I keep a general count of my daily calories, I do not track every calorie I consume. By training my body to eat properly, it now knows what I need and how much and I'm able to trust it more. When I started my Ageless Athlete journey, I couldn't trust my body worth a damn because it had been trained to eat junk. I loved bagels, pizza, hamburgers, chips, cookies, and ice cream. I was a carboholic and the more carbohydrates I ate, the more my body wanted. Sugar had the same effect. I had to go through a withdrawal process to retrain my body. I still have to be careful of the amounts and types of carbohydrates and sugars I eat, but I can certainly allow an occasional splurge. Plus I don't crave junk food anymore and, when I have it, I actually notice what I call a "sugar hangover" the next day and I don't like it very much.

So now you're no doubt asking, "How does the food pyramid work and when and what should I eat?" Since I'm not a nutritionist and there is a plethora of good nutrition books available, getting into too much detail here is beyond the scope of this little book. So, moving on, no doubt your next question is, "Why is eating healthy important for training your Ageless Athlete?" The answer lies in what your body does with the food you eat.

Essentially, the body sees food in one of three categories: carbohydrates, proteins and fats. Each has its role in the body to keep it functioning properly and help it develop as long as you maintain a proper balance of intake. Sounds pretty cryptic, doesn't it. Let's put it in basic terms.

Carbohydrates are fuel for the body. Nutritionists generally recommend that approximately 55 to 60 percent of daily caloric intake be in the form of carbohydrates. As the body absorbs them, they produce glucose in the blood stream, which gives the muscles the energy they need to function. Carbohydrates fall into two sub-categories: simple and complex. The body absorbs simple carbohydrates quicker than complex carbohydrates; therefore, simple carbohydrates tend to be more readily available as a source of energy. If the body doesn't use them, however, or if you eat more carbohydrates than you need for daily activities, your body will convert the excess to fat, which adds mass and weight since fat is stored in the abdomen and under the skin. Complex carbohydrates take longer for the body to absorb, so it has to work harder to do so. They also generally contain ruffage, which the body does not absorb, but is beneficial for cleaning the intestines. Simple carbohydrate sources are sugar and fruits. Complex carbohydrate foods include pasta, bread products, rice, cereal, potatoes, corn and green vegetables such as broccoli and green beans. There are four calories in each gram of carbohydrate.

Since carbohydrates produce glucose, which is fuel for the muscles, the amount of carbohydrates needed to produce the glucose you need for your Ageless Athlete's training activity will depend on your level of muscle use. When I was running my second marathon, I made the mistake of not eating enough the day before and in the early part of the race. By mile 15, I had used up the carbohydrates stored in my muscles, and I started getting tired and a bit lightheaded. This is what is commonly called "hitting the wall." Unfortunately, I didn't know at the time how many carbohydrates I needed to consume pre-race and during the race to avoid or delay "the wall." Luckily, along the race course, my wife gave me a cinnamon raisin bagel, which I ate as I continued to run. My body converted it to glucose and I was able to finish the race. Later, I learned the importance of taking in at least 300 to 400 calories of carbohydrates per hour of training or racing so that my muscles would not deplete the stored glucose as quickly.

Proteins build muscle. As we discussed earlier, muscles get stronger by being stressed during training and then being given time to repair and grow to handle more training stress. Protein is the key ingredient the body uses to build the muscles, which then crave protein to repair the damage done by the training. That is why gyms and fitness clubs sell so many protein supplements. Muscles generally benefit the most when proteins are ingested within an hour after using weights or any other strenuous training. Aside from supplements, major sources of protein include red meats, chicken, pork, fish and, for the vegetarians and those limiting their meat intake, eggs, beans, dairy, and soy products. As with carbohydrates, there are four calories in each gram of protein and nutritionists recommend that 10 to 15 percent of daily caloric intake be in the form of protein foods. As with carbohydrates, excess protein is converted to fat.

The third category the body recognizes is fats, each gram containing a whopping nine calories. The body uses fats for growth and maintenance, insulation against the cold, and energy. Unfortunately, the body doesn't break down stored fats as quickly as carbohydrates to serve as a readily available energy source. That's why many exercise machines that tell you which heart rate range will be for fat burning since the higher ranges, being more intense, will use carbohydrates as the primary energy source. Given the roles of fat (no pun intended) and the high caloric content, as well as the health issues created by excess fat in the body, nutritionists recommend limiting fats to less than 30 percent of daily caloric intake. Generally, there is no reason to focus specifically on eating foods that contain fat since it's already in most of what you eat (other than in green vegetables). The key is to avoid excess fat by eating lean meats, avoiding chicken skin (remember: fat is stored in the skin, even in animals), staying away from fried foods (the oil they are cooked in is full of fats), and limiting snack foods and desserts.

So, to sum up, an Ageless Athlete in training needs to eat enough carbohydrates to provide sufficient energy to train, enough protein to enable the muscles to rebuild and grow, and very little fat. As always, *balance* is the watchword in types and amounts of food, and calorie counting monitors that balance. Use the food pyramid as a guide.

There is one other important nutritional consideration for athletes: free radicals, a byproduct formed when oxygen interacts with certain molecules in the body. These free radicals damage cells and can contribute to aging, heart disease, and cancer. Endurance activities increase the formation of free radicals, so all Ageless Athletes need to take them into account. Although being fit and training regularly will combat the free radicals, eating your fruits and vegetables, particularly the darker colored ones (blueberries, raspberries, strawberries, broccoli, spinach, beets, etc.) helps eliminate them as they form. Fruits and vegetables contain antioxidants that interact with the free radicals and stop them from reacting with other body cells before they can do any damage, so eat at least five servings of fruits and vegetables each day. Blueberries, strawberries, broccoli are among the fruits and vegetables with the highest antioxidant content, but spinach, grapes, carrots, and garlic are also high on the list.

Before going to the next chapter, I want to give you a brief example of this chapter in action. I know a wonderful young woman who for many years was a high-powered professional dedicated to her work to the exclusion of her health. Being relatively short (about five feet), she battled with weight all her life and, unfortunately, until about two years ago, the weight was winning. She was dangerously overweight and in her mid-thirties. One day, her Ageless Athlete finally grabbed her by the shoulders (figuratively speaking) and said, "Enough is enough. You are far too valuable to continue on a course that is killing you slowly." She heard the message, started a BALANCED diet one day at a time, and, that Christmas, asked her father for a treadmill. Her eating regimen followed the formula discussed previously. Now, two years later, she has worn out the first treadmill and now has one that goes faster and has a steeper incline. She gets on it every day before going to work. She has not only lost a major amount of weight, but she has also become more active, self-assured, and, most important, happy with herself. She is an Ageless Athlete and, although she does not compete in any specific athletic, she challenges herself daily to improve her physical conditioning and fitness. She is proud of her accomplishments, and I am too because this wonderful young woman is my daughter.

CHAPTER NINE — A FEW MORE TRAINING TIPS

Know Pain, Know Gain

As your body gets stronger, faster, and fitter from the training process, it is critical that your mind also receive proper training because your mind drives your body. Two key elements are required for training your mind. The first is to be aware of your body's condition and level of performance at all times. The second, which actually derives from the first, is mental toughness. My former Ironman training coach held four Ironman World Championship age group records. He says what distinguishes him from the rest of the field is mental, not physical. In other words, he knows how exactly far he can push his body during training sessions to make himself as fit as possible. Equally important, if not more important, he also learned how to endure pain at a level that matched his body's maximum output. Many athletes are extremely well trained physically, but they don't realize where their bodies' limits are or are unable to endure the pain associated with reaching these limits. My coach pointed out that pushing the body this hard is a tricky and potentially dangerous effort since, if you push too hard or don't know when the pain ceases being good pain and becomes injury-indicating pain, serious negative physical consequences can follow.

My coach is at the extreme end of mental awareness and toughness and well beyond mere mortal Ageless Athletes. I bring this up because this book is primarily for non-elite Ageless Athletes and none of you reading this book has to seek the levels of training or pain that my coach is able to handle. You do need, however, to focus on knowing what your body can and cannot do and how to handle a level of pain that, while it certainly hurts (after all, that's what makes it pain), is a part of pushing the body beyond where it was. OK, you've heard it before, but it's absolutely true: No pain, no gain.

After my hip replacement surgery, I couldn't do any meaningful effort on the stationary cycle for three weeks. During that time, my muscles lost a significant level of fitness. It's an unfortunate byproduct of aging that any hiatus (beyond a week) in training results in an acceleration of loss of fitness. So, when I started trying to rebuild my fitness level, I had to significantly lower the resistance level on the cycle, my pedaling cadence dropped, and my heart rate was way above the level it was when I was training before the layoff. As a result, I had to recognize that my body could only handle a certain level of effort and resistance, and I also needed to accept a certain level of muscle burn and pain to get beyond where I was. I knew my efforts had to be gradual, which required far more patience than I generally possess. My workouts were limited and I needed more recovery time between them than I had previously been used to. But over time, I came back and I still marvel at the process and my Ageless Athlete's almost miraculous ability to re-emerge with a shiny new metal hip joint. Indeed, only four months after my surgery, I was biking 80 miles a week at a faster average speed than I had ever achieved. My layoff gave my body a full rest, which, through the buildup of slow but consistent workouts over several months with gradual intensity increases, enabled me to work up to higher levels than I had previously been able to achieve.

It was a renewal of my Ageless Athlete without specific competitive goals in mind.

There is a concept called periodization in the professional sports training world, which involves periods (usually measured in monthly or bi-monthly intervals) where the athlete focuses on different types of training (for example, long, slow endurance-building, high intensity interval work and specific training toward a given competition). This type of training also requires an off period to give the body and mind time to recover and relax. During this off period, the athlete does no specific training in his or her sport but instead merely does enough general exercise to stay reasonably fit. My recovery from surgery was one of those off periods and, since then, I have attempted to incorporate similar off periods into my yearly training cycles.

Balance, Focus, and Discipline

Training is a **BFD** situation — no, not THAT BFD. I mean **Balance, Focus, and Discipline**. Balance is finding the proper mix of training, recovery, and other things that are important in life. Focus means keeping mentally aware during training of exactly what you're doing, how your body is reacting, and your overall goals. Discipline is making sure the training is consistently done.

Putting unrealistic expectations on ourselves is a major hindrance to Balance. Planning to run a marathon that is only a month or two away, for example, will create serious stress if we are running only 15 miles a week. This stress will push us to set unrealistic daily and weekly training goals which, if not met, will increase the stress and, if met, will increase the risk of injury. In either case, I guarantee the training will become a major chore and will cease being enjoyable. You will have one unhappy Ageless Athlete and you will run the risk of giving up totally or getting injured.

I like to approach training with both realistic short-and longer-term goals. This is a combination of Balance and Focus. The short-term goal could be a short distance race in the near future that serves as a training-level test. The longer-term goal could be a longer-distance race later in the season. Sometimes short-term goals are realistically attainable higher levels of fitness that you can set on a monthly basis. I try to keep Balanced between my short- and long-term goals as I train, using the short-term goals to keep me Focused and the longer-term goals to keep me Disciplined.

A Balance of easy, moderate, and hard training days is necessary during the training process itself. Never put hard days back to back. You need a Balance of stress and recovery. After a hard day, an easy day (or rest day) should follow. For the same reason, don't string too many easy days in a row; otherwise you won't really have anything to recover from.

Also, be aware of bumps in the training so they don't throw you off course. You'll have good days and bad days, for example. Sometimes you'll be "in the zone" with your training or a particular event and the following week, you may fall back miserably. Be aware that the body is not a machine. It is influenced by complex factors both internally and externally. While some self-analysis about why you fell back can lead to valuable learning experiences, you'll still have ups and downs that will not always be explainable.

You might also have to take a forced hiatus from training because of work or some other important life event. Even when these bumps occur, however, most of the time I can still fit in some training even if it is far less often than I'd like or not exactly what I'm used to. That way I keep in touch with my Ageless Athlete and preserve at least a minimum level of Balance, Focus, and Discipline in my training process. I'll probably be a little depressed and more irritable during the hiatus, though, since my endorphin level will be less and my ability to handle stress will likewise decrease. Also, I must mentally prepare myself for the fact that getting back to my training routine will require some extra Discipline once the hiatus is over. But I will "Just do it," as the Nike slogan says, even though I may be unmotivated at first. My Ageless Athlete will quickly come alive again and I'll be happy once I'm back to my normal training routine.

Learn From the Pros

No matter which athletic endeavor you choose, there will always be others who have been doing it longer and have more experience. There are probably professional athletes who are doing it as well, whether it's golf, tennis, mountain climbing, fishing, or bowling. So, read books about your sport or other athletic activity to gain inspiration and motivation from others' experiences and achievements. Watch the pros compete if you have the opportunity. Something they are doing can help you improve your technique or abilities. Remember, however, they are pros and they train extensively every day with sophisticated coaching and training tools. Don't expect to reach their levels; just enjoy the fact that you compete in the same athletic endeavors they do, even if you're not as physically gifted or as young as they are. You are an athlete just like them. Respect your athleticism, regardless of the level you're at, regardless of whether you are the first, in the middle, or dead last. You can continue to improve for the rest of your life. Walk with self-assurance, shoulders back, chin up. Swagger a little if you feel the urge. You've earned it.

Keep a Log

I am a great believer in charting my training. I religiously enter my athletic activity every day in my log. Seeing how much I have actually done over a week, a month, or even a year, gives me a great sense of accomplishment. I can also compare my current data to prior years and as I get older and a bit slower, I can still see that I have not fallen far from where I was several years earlier. Keeping my log also forces me to do my training because I don't want any months with significantly fewer results than prior months and I certainly don't want any year where I haven't maintained at least a base line of training. Regardless of your level of training, your log generates accountability. I am accountable for my training and my health. My log shows me whether I am slacking off and, more importantly, how much progress I've made and how I can sustain that progress.

There are several ways to keep a log: set up a daily diary, buy an athletic training log book (any decent-sized book store will carry several choices) or keep your log on your computer as I do. I joined a website called "Beginner Triathlete," that has a log where I can easily and quickly enter my daily swimming, biking, running, and weight training records. The website keeps a tally of my weekly, monthly, and yearly totals, so it's easy to look back and see my progress over the months. While there's nothing wrong with taking breaks, they can't be too long. I rarely take a full week off but I might shorten my amount per day or be less intense, and I might add in extra days off. But my log keeps me honest since what I do is right there in black and white, so I can't make faulty memory excuses to exaggerate what I think I actually did.

Progress, Not Perfection

Progress is a cornerstone of athleticism. As we have seen, training is progressive because we add new layers of intensity, speed, endurance, skill, or power with each workout to improve at our chosen athletic activity.

Progress is a measured comparison over time. It is seeing where you started and watching yourself move forward. You may have goals along the way, both short-and long-term as previously discussed, but the most important goal is to enjoy the journey. Bob Dylan made a thought-provoking statement in one of his songs: "He not busy being born is busy dying." Even though he probably wasn't thinking of athletics when he wrote that lyric, it certainly applies. As an athlete, your training is a constant growth process. You are born over and over again as your body tears down and rebuilds to a stronger and more fit level to produce a new and improved you each time you train. Training will prolong your life and creative processes. When you regenerate your body, you regenerate your mind as well. That is how strong the mind-body connection is. I bear no ill will toward couch potatoes, but I'm convinced they are busy dying, and I for one prefer to be busy living.

Getting back to my log, I occasionally look back over the years to see how far I've progressed. I'm amazed to see that I'm often better at some things now even though I may be years older. As I mentioned earlier, a few months after my hip replacement surgery, I reached average biking speeds that I never achieved before. That gives me more motivation to keep pushing myself. I never want to say I have done all I can do. It just isn't so.

Finally, do not let your expectations and disappointments undermine your progress. It is the rare individual who wins every event. Actually, it is probably more accurate to say it is the rare individual who wins any event. On any given day, you never know who else is going to show up as your competition. You never know what the weather is going to be and how it will affect your performance. Expecting to win should not be your mindset. Doing your best and being satisfied with the result is a far more realistic goal. Sometimes I feel sluggish, tired, or just plain unmotivated at a race and need to accept that finishing may be the best

I am going to do. But I make it a goal to finish. Then, when I do, I may not be as happy with my results as I have been in other races, but I am not disappointed, frustrated, and upset.

In my second year of competing in triathlons, I did a race in Montauk, New York, where a large number of triathletes from my local triathlon club were also competing. I felt I was well trained and wanted to place in the top three in my age group to show my fellow club members what a good triathlete I was. I looked at the other racers in my age group and figured I could easily pick up third place at least. I finished fourth. I am embarrassed to tell you this, but I was so angry that I refused to attend the after-race festivities and I went off by myself during the awards ceremony — resulting in my not being there to cheer my wife who did place in the top three in her age group and received a medal. I've never forgotten that race, not because of my fourth-place finish, but because it was the low point of my negativity (and immaturity). I was selfish and took all the joy out of competing and being with fellow triathletes and friends. I abandoned my Ageless Athlete that day. But I also learned a valuable lesson about the devastating after effects of my unreal and inappropriate expectations and ego.

PART D

CONCLUSION

CHAPTER TEN — PATTY'S STORY

Up until now this book has focused on your Ageless Athlete in her or his pursuit of an athletic passion. This chapter will show you how your Ageless Athlete can even help save your life. An exaggeration? Read on as my wife, Patty, tells you her story:

Hi. I'm Patty and I'm a cancer survivor. As I write this, I'm completing my training for the New York City Marathon in early November. One year ago, I was diagnosed with Stage IV lung cancer, which had metastasized and traveled to my brain to form an inoperable malignant tumor in addition to the inoperable lung tumor. By all rights, I shouldn't even be here telling you this story, but I don't want to put the cart before the horse, so let me go back in my life and set the stage.

I smoked cigarettes for more than twenty years. Although I was athletic as a child and even in my early adult years, I was also a smoker. I didn't give up the habit until my husband, Charlie, having found his Ageless Athlete, gave up smoking himself and forced me to the chilly garage and innumerable dog walks to indulge in my no-longer-welcome habit. That lasted about two years before I was finally able to say "Enough is enough." July 15, 1994, was the day of my last cigarette and, as Charlie likes to call it, my Ageless Athlete's birthday.

When I was a young woman, and although I was a smoker, I hooked up with some local runners in my hometown of Greenwich, Connecticut, and they actually convinced me to do the New York City Marathon with them. I loved the running and the challenges of training and, being young, I was able to complete the marathon despite the cigarettes. As I got older, however, I gave up the running for a life of cigarettes, work, and weekend partying. When I met Charlie, we were both absorbed in this same lifestyle, so imagine how annoyed I was when his Ageless Athlete moved in and upset all my "fun." He gave up the smoking and the partying and I saw him become happier and happier with his newfound "friend." I figured it wouldn't last but it did. I couldn't believe what I was seeing and I realized I had two choices. I could let him and this Ageless Athlete "friend" of his go their merry way or I could join them. I made the decision to join them by giving up smoking and getting back to running.

Giving up smoking was not easy. I was one of those people who really loved cigarettes and I was emotionally addicted in the worst way. I couldn't wait to light up as soon as I got out of bed in the morning and the last cigarette before going to bed was like a teething ring for a baby. I tried the patch, acupuncture, hypnosis, and just about every other available method to stop. I especially liked the patch because smoking with it on was even better than smoking without it. In the end, I knew the only way I could be successful at staying off the cigarettes was to start running.

So I ran, and I ran, and I ran. Charlie called me the Eveready Rabbit because I just kept going and going. I was blessed with a great endurance ability, which is probably why, as a smoker, I was even able to do the New York City Marathon when I was younger. But, being a bit of a Type A personality (as I think most athletes are), I needed goals. I needed a competitive motivation and there was a marathon in D.C. that fall, called the Marine Corps Marathon, which seemed like a good target. Not to be outdone, Charlie started training for it as well and we both completed that marathon that year (1994) and I beat him. He was a good athlete about it and it didn't take him more than a week before he was willing to talk to me again.

The years went on and Charlie and I trained our Ageless Athletes together. As he mentioned earlier in this book, we ran the 100th Boston Marathon together and he actually had to slow down and stay with me to help me get through it so we could cross the finish line together. Obviously, his Ageless Athlete had reached a new maturity level since he didn't complain or rub it in after the race.

Then his Ageless Athlete decided to take up triathlons and I followed suit since I was a swimmer in high school and I knew how to ride a bike. Because of our shared passion for athletics, our lives together became wonderful and we were enjoying leading active, balanced, and healthy lifestyles. Then my work life changed and I was given a position in sales. Using my Type A personality and channeling my athletic discipline into fifteen-hour, pressure-packed workdays, I started making a lot of money, but my training slipped. I did fewer races and I was tired and irritable most of the time. That lasted about two years before the economy fell apart and I changed to a less-stressful work position. But the damage was done. About a year later came that fateful October 31st.

I was 52 years old. Near the end of October, some unusual coordination issues started showing up. I was eating dinner at a restaurant one evening and I thought I was cutting some food with my knife, but when I looked down, my hand was empty. I had dropped the knife and didn't even know it. Then, later that night, I picked up my mini-dachshund, Maggie, under my left arm to take her up the stairs to bed. All of a sudden, she was on the floor. I had dropped her without feeling it. Luckily she was not hurt but I was frightened.

The next morning, I explained my symptoms to my doctor, who immediately made an appointment for me to have a brain MRI. The MRI showed a brain tumor, which was causing my brain to swell, which in turn was causing the coordination problems. The next thing I knew I was admitted into my local hospital for observation, medication, and more tests.

As you can imagine, both Charlie and I were shocked. Here I was, healthy and active one day, and diagnosed with a brain tumor the next. But that was only the beginning because brain tumors are usually caused by cancer somewhere else in the body. So doctors did a complete CT scan of my body and that was when the other shoe dropped. I will never forget that morning of October 31st, less than 12 hours after I was admitted, when the doctor came into my hospital room with the CT scan results and told me I also had a tumor on my lung, right next to my aorta. I asked him how large it was, and he said about the size of a handball. As if that weren't bad enough, he said it was almost definitely a cancerous tumor, which had metastasized and formed the brain tumor. In that one instant, my life had changed forever and I had no idea at that point how much life I had left.

The doctors did some more tests and, of course, confirmed I had cancer. No one smiled. All my family doctor could say to me was, "I guess you know how serious this is." I did after that. Lung cancer is one of the deadliest forms of cancer and the survival rate is one of the lowest, if not the lowest, of all cancers. Most who survive were diagnosed early enough to remove the tumor before it had metastasized. I was clearly not in that group.

For the next week, the doctor kept me in the hospital while he and his staff tried to stop the brain swelling through medications so I wouldn't have a seizure and while they tried to figure out a game plan. Being an athlete, I knew about game plans. I knew my own strengths and how to apply them to capitalize on my opponent's weaknesses. I didn't feel particularly strong at that moment, however, and

I had no idea if my cancer opponent had any weaknesses at all.

But then Charlie's Ageless Athlete kicked in. Applying the "know your event and your competition" rule from his athletic experience, he researched lung cancer and discovered it does have weaknesses — it's anaerobic and needs sugar and an acidic environment to grow. Because of this fact, many nutritionists view making the body alkaline, and removing sugar from the diet, will starve the cancer and even kill it. Charlie found books about which foods fight cancer and why they work. Natives of India, for example, have only 20 percent of the level of lung cancer that we have in the United States. Nutritionists believe it is related in large part to the spices they eat in their food, particularly turmeric (curcumin). Charlie also discovered the body's own immune system has an amazing power to kill cancerous cells if given the right tools, and that many times throughout our lives, our bodies develop cancerous cells our immune system kills off before they can multiply and spread. He learned that stress tears down our immune systems, giving cancer the opportunity to grow to such a point that we cannot fight back and that cancer, being a cunning and resilient competitor, immediately attacks the weakest organs. In my case, my body was compromised when I was working that stress-filled sales position and, having been a smoker (even though I had given it up 14 years earlier), my lungs became an easy target.

When Charlie told me all this, I was really ticked off! How dare this invader think it could just walk all over me? Now that I knew about my competition and the kind of "training" I needed to fight it, my athletic juices took over. I knew I had to fight back. I realized I needed to do the same kinds of things an athlete does to prepare for a competition.

I also discovered statistics are inherently suspect and not to be relied on. First of all, people have survived Stage IV lung cancer and there was no reason I couldn't be one of them. Second, the statistics don't delve deeply into the underlying details about those who do survive and those who don't, their physical and mental condition at the time of their diagnosis, and what they did or didn't do to fight back. So, I threw the statistics out the window. They don't apply to me and they don't count. I am my only statistic.

All this change in attitude started happening during the week I was in the hospital as doctors tried to stabilize my brain swelling so I would be less likely to have a seizure. They told me that, even after I was released, I wasn't allowed to do any running until the brain swelling decreased sufficiently so that I wouldn't have a seizure. During my hospital stay, I walked around the corridors on the hospital grounds. Because my coordination was still a bit off, Charlie had to keep tilting me to my left side so I would walk straight. I didn't even know I was listing to the left. These walking sessions helped keep me sane and gave me a feeling that I was still functioning. The trouble with a cancer diagnosis is that it has such a big scary reputation, which can produce a paralyzing fear, but I wasn't going to give in to its trash talk hype or intimidating look. With the help of my athlete's mindset and my husband's and friends' support, I was training to beat it, using the walking a starting point.

It's hard to describe the rollercoaster ride of emotions that a cancer diagnosis brings on and, for me, it was critical that I remained disciplined in my thinking and actions. I did not have the luxury of allowing myself to become depressed. I knew that activity fights depression so I had to keep active. Since there were limits on what I was physically allowed to do, Charlie and I started to focus on my game plan. Based on what the doctors were saying, we saw three distinct lines of attack, all of which needed to be undertaken simultaneously. One line of attack was, of course, the medical, but my real efforts would be focused on attacking my cancer through both fitness and nutrition.

The goal was to help my body develop the tools, including enabling my own immune system, to stop the cancer from spreading and cause it to die.

We had to deal with the brain tumor first. As luck (or, as I prefer to think of it, providence) would have it, there was this new amazing machine called a Cyberknife that could kill tumors by zapping them with laser-thin radiation rays that did not harm any surrounding tissue. At the time, there were only about 200 of these machines in existence in the United States, and my hospital had one. Since my brain tumor was located too deep to be surgically removed, the Cyberknife became my only hope.

The Cyberknife procedure consisted of three consecutive daily sessions of lying on a table with a mask tightly over my head and bolted down so I couldn't move while the Cyberknife did its zapping. Each session lasted about an hour and was totally non-invasive with no apparent side effects. The whole Cyberknife process was completed about two weeks after I was released from the hospital. Once the brain tumor was zapped, chemotherapy was the next medical action.

Because I came into this whole mess in otherwise good physical condition (thanks to my training as a triathlete), I was eligible for heavy chemotherapy (lucky me) since the doctors felt I was strong enough to handle it. That meant all-day chemo sessions every three weeks for a cycle of three sessions. Not fun, but I never had any side effects. Throughout the cycle, I was able to go for three-to four-mile walks and, once the brain doctors felt the tumor had disintegrated sufficiently for there to be no more risk of seizure, I was able to start running again. One of the more insidious effects of cancer for me, though, was psychological. Because I had it in my body, my mind was starting to believe I was powerless to do any physical activity. By continuing to exercise, however, particularly when I could run again, I was able to dispel this feeling and replace it with the good feelings that come when endorphins are released through aerobic exercise. I cannot emphasize enough how important my walking and running became for combating my cancer, both physically and psychologically.

During the chemo cycle, nutrition became essential because chemo drugs are poison and wreak havoc with the immune system and other body activities. Unfortunately, I don't believe the medical profession really understands how powerful proper nutrition can be, not only in countering the negative effects of chemotherapy, but also in fighting cancer itself. One of my oncologists told me that, in medical school, she was only required to take one course on nutrition. So I knew I was going to have to forge my own way on this line of attack even though my oncologists did support my efforts.

Charlie embarked on an expansive research project regarding the relationship between what we eat and cancer. I was always a reasonably healthy eater but I must admit I did like my steak and ice cream (not together of course). Since cancer thrives on sugar and is anaerobic, the goal for me was to remove all sugar (other than the natural sugar in fruits and vegetables) from my diet and make my body alkaline (which is aerobic and not anaerobic). This meant essentially a diet of vegetables, fruit, fish, and some chicken, with no bread, rice, pasta, processed foods, or red meat. Since there were many reports about turmeric and hot freshly brewed green tea being major cancer-fighting foods, they also became a staple of my diet. I put the turmeric in olive oil with black pepper (since the pepper is needed for our bodies to absorb the turmeric) and used it as my salad dressing. It is amazing how not wanting to die motivated me to give up things I never would have given up otherwise, and eat things I never would have eaten in a lifetime.

We also found a nutritionist who specialized in bolstering the immune system and he prescribed a raw fruit and vegetable diet with specific nutrition supplements. I also met Walter Levine, an entrepreneur and multiple myeloma cancer survivor, who introduced me to another nutritional supplement called TBL-12, which is composed of sea cucumber and some other sea-related ingredients. Apparently, the sea cucumber's immune system is compatible with our own and actually bolsters our ability to fight cancer. A hospital in New York City is even conducting a clinical trial on TBL-12 using multiple myeloma cancer patients. I started taking the TBL-12 immediately and have not stopped since.

Within the first three months of being diagnosed, my Stage IV lung cancer did not spread any further and the lung tumor actually shrank enough that surgery became an option. I don't know for sure whether chemotherapy, mental toughness, physical fitness, raw diet, or TBL-12 was the primary contributor or whether it was the combination of all of them, but my oncologist was able to set me up with one the best lung tumor surgeons at Mass General in Boston. The weekend before we went to Boston, I did a 5K running race, sponsored by the Susan B. Komen Foundation, which raises money to fight breast cancer. I didn't know if this race would be my last ever, so I wanted to race for a worthy cause.

In the first week of February, Charlie and I flew to Boston for the surgery. The surgeon informed us, however, that removing the tumor was still only a possibility because of my advanced stage of cancer. Ultimately, he couldn't make a decision whether to remove the tumor until he removed and biopsied the lymph nodes around my windpipe. If the cancer showed up in any of these lymph nodes, he would call off the surgery because it would not do me any good. If no cancer showed up, he would proceed with the surgery without predicting whether he could actually remove the tumor or all of the cancer. The tumor was very close to my aorta, so what he saw when he went in determined whether the surgery was too risky. Certainly not the most encouraging surgical prognosis I could have ever heard, but I wanted the cancer out, so the surgery was scheduled for two days later.

When I woke up in the recovery room, the first thing I asked was how long I had been in the operating room. I knew if I had only been there a couple of hours, the surgeon would not have removed the tumor. Turns out I had been in for about six hours. Not only did the surgeon remove the tumor, but he also removed the lung tissue around it, biopsied a large number of lymph nodes, and removed all the cancer he could find. I lost half my left lung in the process but, as far as I was concerned, that was a small price to pay to get rid of the tumor.

When I returned home, I was still weak but I was determined to walk every day, even if for only 10 minutes, to begin rebuilding my stamina. But because I was coughing a lot from the surgery, I could only do a little at a time. Gradually as the weeks rolled by, I was able to walk as much as three miles at a time. I might have been able to do more but my oncologist put me through another chemo cycle as a precautionary measure.

Because of the lung surgery and the increased potency (and deadliness) of this precautionary round of drugs, I was far more tired from this round of chemo than I was the first, so I did not make much progress in my walking even though I still kept it up at least five days a week. I knew I needed to continue to hold onto my athleticism. It had become a core part of who I am and a key factor in my battle against cancer. Plus, I loved it and was not going to let the cancer or the chemo take it away from me.

Throughout the additional round of chemo, I never gave up my thought of running the New York City Marathon and, once the chemo ended and I started recovering more energy, I was actually able to add some short-run intervals into my walks and extended the walking to four, then five, miles. By the time June 1st came, I was committed to doing the marathon.

Although I had trained for several marathons in the past, with only three quarters of my lungs, I had no idea how much training I could handle. Charlie worked out a plan where I would combine running and walking intervals into increasingly longer distances with the length of the run intervals increasing each week. My last long run/walk was 19 miles, about 16 of which was running. This training program is not as aggressive as it would be for someone trying to achieve a specific pace and time for a marathon, but my goal was to finish tired, but standing, happy and still healthy. I wanted to show other cancer victims that it can be done. We all know that Lance Armstrong has proved this, but many, if not most, cancer victims think he is something of a phenomenon and far beyond mere mortal abilities. I am one of those mere mortals one who hopes and believes we all have a little Lance in us. With our Ageless Athletes, no doors are closed to us and a full and active life is available. To prove this, I will finish the New York City Marathon both for myself and anyone else who wants to hope and believe. Look for me on TV — I will be the woman wearing the shirt that says:

"I Am a Stage IV Lung Cancer Survivor."

***

Patty finished the New York City Marathon in five hours and five minutes, which placed her in the middle of the finishers — an amazing ending to an amazing story and I can think of no better way to end this book.

I wish all of you the full lifetime of rewards that my Ageless Athlete has brought me and that your Ageless Athlete can bring you. I hope this little book has given you the belief and motivation to find the Ageless Athlete that lies within each of us, waiting for the opportunity to motivate you to pursue your passion and bring the many rewards that will follow. God bless.

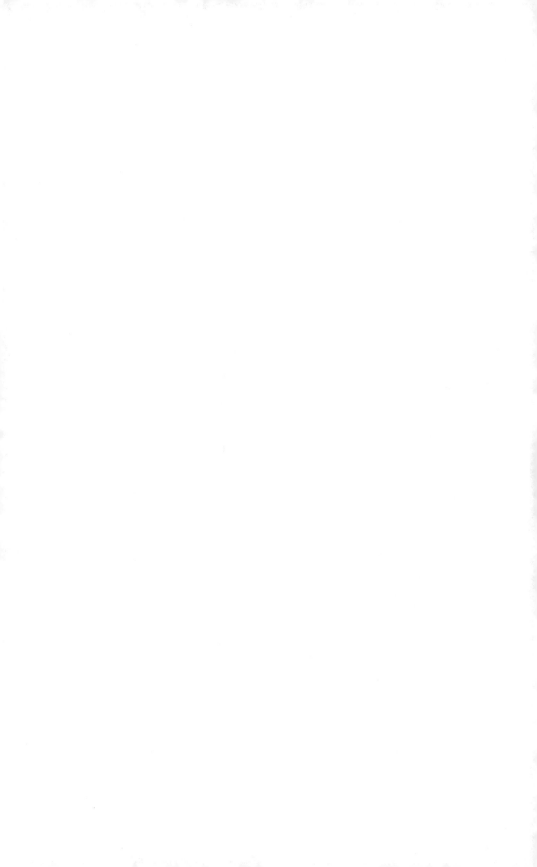

Printed in the United States
By Bookmasters